One of the best indicators of clinical success is the empathy of the clinician. Although not trained as clinical psychologists, the Davises have loads of empathy for the plight of the infertile. The insights expressed in *Infertility's Anguish* can help you move past the pain and into action and acceptance.

— Michael E. Young, Ph.D., Assistant Professor of Psychology,
   Southern Illinois University at Carbondale

Infertility's Anguish helps couples to face and cope with the emotional issues of infertility. It can improve communication between a husband and wife, allowing them to deal with infertility's challenges as a more cohesive unit than before.

— Printha Merritt, Facilitator of Silent Angels,
   a church sponsored infertility support group

For those who know the sadness and hopelessness couples experience with infertility, Jan & Dan's book *Infertility's Anguish* offers, with compassion, love, and understanding, a ray of hope at the end of a dark tunnel.

— Ciro J. Rustici, Doctor of Chiropractic, Independence, Missouri

Infertility's Anguish

Everyone *Else* Is Pregnant, Why Not *Us*?

Jan & Dan Davis

Second Star Creations

Infertility's Anguish - Everyone *Else* is Pregnant, Why Not *Us*?
By Jan & Dan Davis

This book is not intended as a remedy for infertility's medical or emotional issues. Infertility is extremely complicated; we recommend professional medical or emotional help if you believe you need it.

Published by: Second Star Creations
12120 State Line Rd #190, Leawood, KS 66209-1254
http://www.secondstar.us
Email to: ordersIA@secondstar.us

Cover by Matthew Armstrong
Author Photo by Karl Wiedamann

All rights reserved. No part of this book may be reproduced or transmitted in any form or by any means, electronic or mechanical, including photocopying, recording, or by any information storage or retrieval system, without written permission from the authors, except for the inclusion of brief quotations in a review.

Copyright © 2004 by Jan & Dan Davis
Printed in the United States of America
First Edition

10 9 8 7 6 5 4 3 2 1

Publisher's Cataloging-in-Publication
(Provided by Quality Books, Inc.)

Davis, Jan, 1955-
   Infertility's anguish : everyone else is pregnant, why not us? / Jan & Dan Davis. -- 1st ed.
   p. cm.
   LCCN 2003093561
   ISBN 0-9725977-3-5

   1. Infertility--Popular works. 2. Infertility--Psychological aspects. I. Davis, Dan, 1957- II. Title.

RC889.D33 2004   362.1'96692
                           QBI03-200517

Dedicated to

Shawn, Michelle, and Christy

How to Read This Book

Your inclination may be to read this book from the beginning through to the end. That's how we read most books and that is how you can read this book. However, we realize that many readers like to skim and get the points that are most relevant to them as quickly as possible.

We wrote this book with that in mind. Each of the twenty-five topics consists of two sections, a conversational discussion of the topic and a fictional anecdote, representing the thoughts, feelings, experiences and hopes of the couples we have interviewed.

We have tried to keep each segment as a stand-alone work that you can read without reading other sections of the book.

Because we constructed the book this way, a straight-through reading may cause you to say, "Hmm. They said this already." That will sometimes be true, but in repeating ourselves we have tried to show a slightly different aspect of a given issue.

So please pick a topic.

Read what you want, in whatever order pleases you.

Foreword

The infertility journey is one that I am familiar with as a practicing reproductive endocrinologist of many years. It has been my privilege to become acquainted with many couples making that journey. It is a difficult time in a couple's life and the stress that results is comparable to the stress from other major medical issues such as the diagnosis of cancer.

Jan and Dan honored this truth with their title, *Infertility's Anguish*. Their recommendations, as they describe the progression through infertility diagnosis, treatment and resolution, are practical and heartfelt. Their life experience with infertility and those experiences of the many couples they interviewed for this book have been distilled into advice that is accessible to you.

Infertility's Anguish gives you the chance to glean a perspective on a difficult life stage and gain some control wherever you are in your journey. If you are a friend or family member of someone who is infertile, this book allows you to understand the feelings of couples in the throes of this crisis and recommends how best to *help*. The stories about particular couples were, to me, most helpful in bringing home both the anguish and the hope that is involved in this infertility journey.

I agree wholeheartedly with Jan and Dan's philosophy that infertility, while grueling and filled with disappointments, can be an opportunity for personal growth and a strengthening of your relationship. One of my personal heroines, Dr. Joan Borysenko, has described how major life crises can bring about personal wisdom in her book, *Fire in the Soul: A New Psychology of Spiritual Optimism*.

I have had the opportunity to observe many couples travel through this difficult time and have seen the great joy that comes with having a biologic child. I have also seen many other wonderful families grow from donor eggs or sperm and adoption. These options may not have been considered at the beginning of the struggle for parenthood, but were arrived at after working through the grief of initial failures.

Some couples choose to remain childfree and reclaim their former sense of confidence by taking their other life plans off hold, such as returning for an advanced degree.

While it has always been my first goal to assist the couple in my care to have a child, I have always hoped that I can offer guidance to them so that they arrive at the end of their infertility journey with the ability to return to the rest of their lives with selves intact and a desire to live to the fullest. I believe Jan and Dan have written this book in that loving spirit.

Dr. Jennifer Thie
Reproductive Endocrinologist
Cincinnati, Ohio
July 2003

Contents

Dedication 5
How to Read This Book 6
Foreword 7
Preface 11

Part 1 - Realizing There's a Problem 13

Are We Infertile? 15

Do We Keep Quiet or Tell the World? 29

Have We Done Something Wrong? 37

Why Doesn't My Family Understand? 47

Why Does the Man Care? 55

How Do We Keep Communicating? 69

Part 2 - Trying to Get Pregnant 77

Seeking Help, Choosing a Doctor 79

Handling Drugs and Surgery 91

Examining Alternative Pregnancies 103

Considering Prayer 111

Part 3 - Acknowledging Your Emotions 119

Riding the Roller Coaster 121

Never Expect to be in Control 127

Oh, Those Holidays 133

What We've Lost 141

Contents

Part 4 - Dealing with Your Emotions   149

    Sharing Your Pain with Others   151

    Handling What People Say   161

    Staying in Touch with Your Spouse   173

    Dealing with Work   183

    Accepting Others' Parenting Decisions   197

    Giving Love to Pets   201

Part 5 - Moving on with Your Life   207

    Coping Mechanisms   209

    Naming an Unborn Child   215

    Adoption as an Option   221

    Childless or Childfree?   231

    What We've Gained   239

Afterword   247

    Ode to Shawn   250
    From Our Children, Who Have Gone Before Us   251
    Acknowledgements   252
    About the Authors   253
    About Second Star Creations   254

Preface

If you've picked up this book, you are probably in a lot of pain, stress and sorrow, or you know someone who is. We want to tell you that you are not alone. Knowing you are not alone won't help you get pregnant, but it will help make your daily struggle with infertility a little easier.

During our own infertility journey, we felt alone. Bookstores had books on how to get pregnant, but we found very few that dealt with how we were feeling. All the books appeared to assume that if you did exactly what they told you to do, you would get pregnant, rarely addressing the pain and emotional anguish infertility entails.

Today, some of the medical texts on infertility now include a chapter or two on how it feels to be infertile. Occasionally, you will find a book addressing the emotional issues, usually from the woman's point of view. Helpful organizations like RESOLVE, the National Infertility Association, and other local groups continue to grow and reach out to infertile couples. We heartily applaud these efforts. Everything that helps us understand what we are going through can make the infertility struggle a little easier.

As an infertile couple, we believe how infertile couples feel should be shared and that both the man's and woman's viewpoints should be explored. Both go through infertility, although in different ways. We interviewed numerous couples in researching this book, but not as a doctor or psychologist analyzing the situation. We've lived this journey for many years.

Writing this book was slow going. Dan left two jobs to take some time to write, since he didn't seem to have time during his work. We persevered, because we felt a book like this had to be written. It is the book we wanted to buy during our infertility struggle. It doesn't deal with the medical aspects of how to get pregnant; there are many good books on that subject.

Instead, through conversations and fictional anecdotes, we illustrate the emotions an infertile couple experience. Starting with the earliest realization of infertility, we move into medical treatment, and then explore the emotions that come with the struggle and how to deal with them. Finally, we discuss how to cope day-to-day, including the choice of adoption versus living childfree.

There are no magical answers in this book. We wish there were! Our hope is that the book can at least help you to better understand yourself and your spouse's feelings when dealing with this issue. In understanding yourself, you will be better able to make choices that will enrich your life and make your life as good as it can be under the circumstances you are dealing with.

Most of all, we hope you can have the child you desire. We hope this book will eventually gather dust on your bookshelf, because you only needed it for a short time.

Unlike the medical texts, however, which you should never need again, this book can be pulled out, years later, and you can say, "Yes, indeed, this is how I felt. This is what I went through. In reading *Infertility's Anguish*, I realized that I was not alone. That, in itself, helped me make it through each day until I finally had my child."

If we can accomplish that, our time spent writing this book will have been worthwhile.

Dan T. Davis
Janet L. Lazo-Davis
October 2003

Part 1
Realizing There's a Problem

Are We Infertile?
    Realizations   15
    Rude Awakenings   19

Do We Keep Quiet or Tell the World?
    Do I Want to Be Alone?   29
    You Are Not Alone   33

Have We Done Something Wrong?
    The Sin of Infertility   37
    Children Are Required   43

Why Doesn't My Family Understand?
    Related Opinions   47
    A Test of Wills   51

Why Does the Man Care?
    Life Goes On   55
    The Story of G'Nor   61

How Do We Keep Communicating?
    Honesty: The Best Medicine   69
    What's So Funny?   73

Statistic on the back cover is estimated based on data in the report:
Abma J, Chandra A, Mosher W, Peterson L, Piccinino L.
Fertility, family planning, and women's health: New data from the 1995 National Survey of Family Growth.
National Center for Health Statistics. Vital Health Stat 23(19).
1997.

RESOLVE, the National Infertility Association, is referenced throughout this book. They can be reached at http://www.resolve.org.

— Are We Infertile? —

Realizations

Welcome to the infertility journey. All of us are reluctant members of this traveling group. If at any point, you are able to leave us, please do so. We will happily wave you on to your freedom as we continue down the path, hoping that some day we too can leave the road of infertility.

Infertility? Who fits in such a group?

Many of us do. We apply the definition of infertility to any couple that is not able to conceive a child, give birth to a child, or have a child that lives past infancy. Consider the scenarios below:

- A couple has decided they would like a child and has unprotected sex for a year. No pregnancy occurs. They now start dealing with the precise timing of cycles and worry whether medication or surgery will be necessary to correct the problem.

- A woman has no trouble getting pregnant, but she can't carry to term. She and her husband endure one or several miscarriages, never having a baby.

- A woman has a medical issue (endometriosis, tubal pregnancy, etc.) that leaves her with permanent damage to her reproductive systems. Or a man is sterile.

- A couple has a child, but cannot seem to have another.

The group of people who can call themselves infertile is large and the causes of infertility are varied. The only ticket to admission is the desire for a child that you cannot seem to have.

We are at the beginning of this infertility journey. Let's explore together the trials and tribulations that we may have to experience. Together, because the main point of this book is that we are not traveling alone; there are many who walk this road.

Few of us start out with the idea that we might be infertile, or have trouble having children. Even when you are a young child, there is an expectation in our society that some day you will have children.

As children, we play at being either a mommy or a daddy. Admittedly, the **Daddies** are often forced into the role by the **Mommies**, but that only serves to emphasize how society places us in our roles at an early age. Even in single parent families or extended families the concept is passed on to children that *big people* have and raise *little people*.

When you get old enough to realize how little people come about, you also realize that you can have one. The concept that you cannot have one is rarely considered. If you decide to be sexually active before marriage, the idea of becoming pregnant or making someone pregnant is scary. It's not time yet to have children, but engaging in sex opens up the idea that it might happen.

Thus, as we grow up, most of us perceive ourselves as able to have children, and either ignore it, deal with it through preventive measures, or abstain from sex because it could lead to having children.

There are many forces in society that teach us we can have children; in fact, many believe it is somewhat of a God-given right.

Since it is such a fundamental expectation, some of us delay having children until our late twenties or thirties. Why not? Since we can choose when to have a family, we will certainly be able to say: "We decided to wait to have kids until I was twenty-eight. Then we decided to get pregnant with little Jimmy."

We expect that having little Jimmy will be just as planned an event as getting married, going to college, or deciding what to have for dinner.

Realizing There's A Problem

Realizing that you are infertile usually comes gradually, rather than suddenly or violently. Even so, it still comes as a surprise. Finding out that you are infertile is not much different than being diagnosed as having a debilitating disease, realizing you can't find a new job quickly, or determining that a loved one is exhibiting signs of Alzheimer's.

In any of these situations, the natural reaction is one of denial: "This isn't supposed to happen to me." It is a shift from the expected, a realization that we are going to have to deal with something that we never thought of having to deal with.

Infertility is an insidious realization; one that grows within us over time, as we either fail to get pregnant, or find ourselves unable to bring a child to term. For some couples a quick and accurate diagnosis may result in a faster realization of the problem, but still, one has to get to the point where a diagnosis is sought. Others simply continue to *try*, and wonder more and more what is wrong, but refrain from getting a diagnosis. And for some couples, children simply don't arrive, and no doctor can say exactly why.

The teenage years of worrying about having children, or even the early married years of worrying about having children too soon, suddenly shift into "Why aren't we having children?"

After a time, this becomes a nagging worry. And then a strange fear that sits in the pit of your stomach each time you or your spouse (or your significant other) has a menstrual period.

Soon a period becomes a death knell that occurs every month or so, depending on your regularity. It becomes a death in the sense that you have not produced new life, regardless of how hard you tried. It is a symbol of failure. It is a statement that you have once again failed at something that you have always been told is not only normal, but easy to do. Meanwhile, all of your friends, relatives, and co-workers are having children. Everyone else is pregnant. Everyone else has kids!

Insidiously, infertility has crept into your life. At some point, the denial disappears, and you perceive yourself as infertile.

As different from others.

Whether you like it or not, you are now in a new group of people you never thought you'd belong to. Often you feel that you are alone in that category, because just as you are hesitant to share your problems; so are others in the group.

But you are not alone.

Knowing that doesn't change your situation, but maybe it can help you understand your reactions to the fact that you are unable to have a child and deal with it better. We have now embarked on our journey down the road of infertility.

In numbers there can be strength.

— Are We Infertile? —

Rude Awakenings

"Let's have a baby!" Tammy announced happily as we walked through the park. I was carrying a small rock maple sapling and a half-shovel as she said this, and right then I stepped on a root and stumbled, losing the shovel and almost dropping the maple.

"It's not that bad of an idea," she continued, as she handed me the shovel and pretended to brush me clean. I hadn't really fallen to the ground.

Actually, it wasn't a bad idea. I had been entertaining the thought myself, and on a day like today, everything seemed alive, even with the leaves on the trees just beginning to change color.

It was a beautiful late summer Labor Day festival. The park service had just opened up a fairly barren section of land and named it Arbor Fest Woods. To allow the public to participate in its creation, they had been invited to plant a tree in this new section for a small fee. It wasn't difficult to do because they had already dug the designated holes. All you had to do was to pick the hole in the area you wanted, drop the sapling in place, and cover the hole with the dirt that was next to it with the half shovel.

As we walked, everything I saw seemed to challenge the autumn that was coming. We were carrying a new tree, it was absolutely perfect weather, and small children were making happy noises as they ran around the park. It was only natural to think of having a child our own.

Probably what had prompted Tammy's statement, though, was that her younger sister, Debbie, had announced she was pregnant about three weeks earlier. Tammy and I were both twenty-four, and had been married for almost three years. Debbie had just gotten married the previous spring, and at twenty-one was bubbling about her pregnancy. It hadn't affected Tammy that Cathy, her older sister, had two kids, or that my sister Joan had three. Both of them had seemed enough older so that they were supposed to have kids, whereas we were still planning on them.

Tammy and I seem to plan everything. It isn't fun for us if we haven't figured out what we want to do. We were high school sweethearts, we thought alike, and it was always fun to be around each other because we liked doing the same things. Both of us felt that college was a necessity; so we held off getting married till our junior year when we finally decided we could get by in the married section of the dorms.

After graduation, we both found jobs in our respective areas; I did environmental lab work for a soils testing company, and Tammy started teaching math at the local middle school. We were able to afford a nice apartment near both our jobs, but kids were a definite no-no on the budget. So birth control pills became a requirement.

We scrimped and saved, and even managed to take a wonderful trip to the Grand Canyon on our second anniversary last spring. Both of us love our work, so we couldn't imagine that things could get much better, other than the fact that wanting a family did begin to nag at us both.

We've always both loved kids. Uncle Roger and Aunt Tammy are favorites whenever we visit Cathy's and Joan's. So, it was only natural that we wanted children ourselves.

As we placed the maple in the ground, all of this came together in my mind. It *was* time. We had a little bit in savings, even after taking our trip, and I think that Tammy was ready to leave the school after this year. So even the timing would be perfect if she became pregnant in the next couple of months.

I patted the ground around the tree with the shovel, looked at Tammy, and said, "Yes Let's!"

Laughingly, she planted a big kiss on my cheek and danced around the little sapling.

It was a perfect late summer day.

The birth control pills went by the wayside, and our sexual play was actually enhanced because we were *making a baby* instead of just making love.

It didn't take long for us to announce to the world that we were going to be next in line for the baby train. Tammy would pat Debbie's still flat tummy and announce that Debbie's baby would probably have a playmate, or I would start talking about playing with my kids in addition to playing with my nieces and nephews.

Autumn went by quickly as both of us stayed busy at work. We didn't expect to get pregnant right away — we expected it might take a few months before we hit it right.

But one thing did change. We started going house hunting, even though we didn't have enough extra savings for a down payment. It just seemed natural to think about getting a house, because soon we were going to be a *family*, instead of just a *couple*.

Right before Thanksgiving, Tammy and I saw a new house for sale in our favorite neighborhood. It was one we had actually looked at a couple of times from the outside, even though it wasn't for sale, because it was cute and had a nice yard. It needed a little touch-up paint on the outside, but since I've always liked that kind of work, that didn't bother me.

We called our real estate agent, who arranged for us to see the house the Tuesday before Thanksgiving. The house wasn't big, but it did have three nice bedrooms, and the master had a bath of its own, something we really wanted. What really floored us though was that even though all the bedrooms had doors into the hallway, the master had an extra door into bedroom two. So, it was through this door that we first saw the second bedroom.

It was perfect. It was small and cozy, and decorated in pastels. The upper wall was decorated with Pooh characters with balloons floating all around them. This was clearly the Baby's Room. It was several seconds before my mind registered on the furniture — a small sewing table, a single bed, and a small desk with a computer monitor and keyboard.

"I think the folks living here have been planning to redecorate the room," apologized our real estate agent. "But it's perfect," said Tammy astonished. Once again, the two of us had obviously been thinking the exact same thing, and I couldn't resist giving her a one-armed hug.

Afterwards, we went over our finances. We thought the house was a little bit overpriced and were sure we could get it for less, but even assuming that, the lack of a sufficient down payment was a problem. We could afford the monthly payment; we just couldn't get in the door.

Thanksgiving came and went, school stayed busy for Tammy, and my work continued to be interesting. Christmas suddenly whooshed upon us, and it was time for the family to get together for the big Christmas Eve get-together.

This was always a big deal. Almost all of us lived within thirty minutes of each other, so it wasn't that we didn't see each other during the year. But it was rare that everyone was together in one place. My parents and Tammy's parents lived within two blocks of each other and had been friends when Tammy and I dated, so our families had combined for this event after we were married. This bash always included my parents, Joan and Gary's family, Tammy and me, Tammy's parents, Cathy, Bill and their kids, and this year Debbie was there with her husband, Tony.

Debbie was the hit of the day. She was showing, and everyone commented on it. Debbie was glowing from all the attention, and Tony looked pretty happy about it, too. Debbie told Tammy that she'd adore being pregnant, "Well, at least up until the end of the fifth month." Nope, Tammy admitted, she hadn't had morning sickness, and a lot of discussion ensued about pregnancies and births.

After games with the kids and a big dinner, we settled down to open our presents. The holiday became perfect when we were interrupted by a shout of "It's snowing!" from Daniel, Joan and Gary's oldest, and the large bay window was suddenly covered with lots of face smears from everyone staring outside.

Realizing There's A Problem

It was getting near the end of the presents; Debbie and Tony had even received several for their baby. As I looked over our loot while Tammy and Debbie were gabbing, I noticed that every gift Tammy and I had received had been a gag, whereas everyone else had received nice gifts in addition to the traditional gag gift.

But, before I had time to think any further, Tammy's Dad, who was handing out the gifts, announced, "What have we here?"

A hush fell over the room, and everyone's attention was directed toward Tammy and me. "It looks like a present for Tammy's and Roger's baby!"

Well, no, we weren't pregnant yet; I hadn't left that out of the story. But most everyone knew we were going to be pregnant soon, we hadn't kept that a secret.

It was a small present, and Tammy's Dad made a point of giving it to me, even though Tammy was huddled next to me on the couch. "What is it?" questioned one of the kids, but they were quickly hushed by my Dad.

Embarrassed at all the attention I opened the gift with Tammy. It looked like just a piece of paper. No, it was a check, and the check was for six thousand dollars!

We were floored. Then Debbie chimed in, "It's for your house, silly! Tony and I don't have enough money for a house, but we figured if we all chipped in, and you combined most of your savings with it, you could get that cute little house you've been mooning over for the past month."

Tammy started crying, and I had a few tears in my eyes, too, as hugs were exchanged all around.

As we left, my Dad chided me with a, "Well, son, we wanted to make sure that baby of yours has a decent roof over its head, but you and Tammy better get to work on the other side of the deal, if you know what I mean." We both laughed and bid everyone a "Merry Christmas" as we went back to our apartment.

It was a perfect Christmas.

We moved on Valentine's Day. The Baby's Room looked even better now that it was empty of the office furniture. Tammy had made the room sparkle; it was ready and waiting. We had placed in it only the few baby furniture donations from family members. Maybe we were jumping the gun a little, but it *was* a Baby's Room, and we didn't want it looking like we'd seen it at Thanksgiving.

Admittedly we were getting a little antsy. Six months had come and gone, and nothing had happened. We even began to check into when we should have sex, to increase the chances we'd get pregnant.

Having Debbie around didn't help. She was about seven months pregnant and loving it. I know she had our best interests at heart, and would come over with a new item for our baby's room, because she had bought an identical item to go into the second bedroom in her and Tony's apartment.

Winter ended, and spring roared in like a lion. You can't really dwell on things, and we had our day to day activities to keep us going. Tammy went on a field trip across state in March with her eighth graders for almost a week, and I think both of us were a little upset because it was right when Tammy would be able to get pregnant. I contemplated showing up at the camp just because of that, but realized that was sort of a dumb idea.

Debbie had her baby on April 6. It was a bouncing baby boy, 7 lbs., 2 oz. that they named Michael. As we gathered to celebrate, Debbie whispered to Tammy, "Now it *is* your turn." Tammy didn't laugh. We had recently stopped laughing at comments like that.

It was strange how we had started to dwell on getting pregnant. Our job and our families continued to occupy most of our time, but everything seemed to start pointing to pregnancy, babies, and families. Every TV show, commercial or newspaper article seemed to be about kids or having kids.

After a nice sermon about motherhood on Mother's Day, Tammy was extremely quiet. After lunch, she cleaned the dishes, and went into the Baby's room. She vacuumed the floor, put fresh sheets on the crib, even though the ones there were not dirty, turned out the lights, and closed both doors. I didn't say a word. She didn't go back in the room after that for quite a while.

It had not been a perfect spring.

Ten months! It wasn't supposed to take this long. The Father's Day softball game was coming up, and for the first time since I was a kid, I was dreading it. Luckily, I was still young enough that it was still me and my father who played in the game, but a lot of my friends already had little boys with plastic bats and ball caps on the sidelines.

Tammy seemed in a good mood. She knew I had always enjoyed playing in these games. I had even won a couple with a last-inning home run, or by driving in the winning run. And so it was that, once again, we were in the ninth inning, and losing by one run. My Dad was on third base and there were two outs. I came up to bat, and Jimmy Johnson was catching. He had a habit of trying to make players lose their concentration by talking to them while they were at bat. I never fell for that tactic and would concentrate on the ball, and wouldn't talk to him, at least not while we were playing.

"Hey, didja see how my wife Jenny fixed up our twins? Braves uniforms and everythin'. I tell ya, it's hell having two at once, but when they get fixed up like that, it just makes it all worth while, huh?"

"STRIKE ONE!"

"I hear your sister-in-law Debbie just had one. Is she here? Did she come to see you play? Where's her new baby?"

"BALL ONE!"

"Hey, you and Tammy are about ready to have a family, right? I saw that new house of yours. Pretty cool! How much did you pay for that sucker?"

"BALL TWO!"

"Haven't the two of you been trying for a while? Is Tammy pregnant yet? Is that her over in the stands? How's her school going? Is it nice having her off for summer vacation?"

"FOUL BALL! STRIKE TWO!"

"Come on, level with me. Practicing is sure fun, isn't it? But, I wonder, do you think you're shooting blanks?"

"STRIKE THREE!"

My Dad came to me from third base; he put his arm around my shoulder and comforted me saying "You can't hit the winning run in every year."

When we got home, Tammy decided to go over to Debbie's and see Michael. While she was gone, I went into the still closed-door Baby's Room and turned on the light switch. Christopher Robin was dancing on the switch plate. I looked up at a Pooh who seemed to be saying "Oh, bother." I sat down in the old wood rocker and cried.

It was not a good summer.

It was the beginning of August, and Tammy was getting ready to commit to the next school year. She wasn't on continuing contract, so during the early summer we had been hinting that she wouldn't be coming back since she was going to have a baby. But as the summer dragged on, we started hinting the opposite to the school board, and today was the day she was going in to sign her yearly contract for teaching.

Being the dutiful husband, I went into the office with her and waited for her to do her thing. Most of the conversation went in one ear and out the other, but I picked up on the conversation when I heard the office secretary say, "It's amazing, what happens these days!"

"Yes?" said Tammy.

"You remember Doris Grayson, don't you? She was in your class."

Realizing There's A Problem

"Oh, yes, cute little fourteen year-old. Blonde, curly hair, with a little perky nose?" Tammy responded. I also remembered her; from the times I had visited Tammy's class when I was off on certain afternoons. She was the one who always sat in the front row and asked the most pointed questions about "why was math like that."

"She went off and got pregnant this summer!" stated the office secretary flatly.

"What? Really? Doris?" Tammy stammered.

I could tell she was beginning to lose her composure, so I got up, and said, "Are you done with the paperwork?"

"Oh, yes, we're just talking, now," said the secretary, oblivious to what was happening to Tammy.

When we got into the car, Tammy broke down. I knew she had just had her period a couple of days earlier, and that in itself had become a traumatic revelation for us each month. "Why can't we get pregnant?" she hissed between her sobs.

"Maybe we should see a doctor other than your gynecologist," I suggested quietly.

"He says everything's fine," she declared in a monotone. "And anyway, you've only been trying for less than a year, and sometimes it just takes time. You're only twenty-five, you've got lots of time." she said, imitating her gynecologist's singsong voice. "Anyway, school starts again next week, and I've got lots to do to get ready for that."

I was wondering if it would be a good autumn.

It was Labor Day. I don't know why we did it, and I still don't know if it was a good idea, but we decided to go to the new section of the park where we had planted a tree the year before. We hadn't been back since then. A lot had happened in the previous year.

As we walked through the older area of the park toward the newer section, Tammy exclaimed happily, "Look! The trees! They've grown so much in the past year."

I had to admit, they weren't monsters, but compared to last year, this almost pasture-like area was now populated by trees that were obviously much bigger than they had been the year before.

"Let's go see ours!" Tammy seemed unstoppable as she ran toward the section we'd picked out for our tree. I didn't know why she was so excited, but I laughed and ran to catch up.

I caught up to Tammy and grabbed her shoulders with my hands. I was going to embrace her, but I realized that she was stiff as stone. She shrugged me away. I looked beyond her at our spot. The tree wasn't there. There wasn't even a trace of it. We hadn't misplaced the site; other evidence pointed distinctly at the spot where there was only grass growing. The tree had obviously not even survived the winter, and had long since been replaced by newly sewn grass.

Tammy fell to her knees and started sobbing uncontrollably. I didn't know what to do. Other people were noticing; all I could do was go to my knees as well and try to hold her and calm her. As she was sobbing, I could hear her mutter over and over between sobs, "Why? Why? Why? Why?"

It was not hard to see the symbolism. The tree was her baby. It had been a year, and nothing had happened. Nothing! We had done all the right things, even to the point of starting to make *sure* we were doing the right things.

Now what?

— Do We Keep Quiet or Tell the World? —

Do I Want to Be Alone?

If you are reading this book, you (or someone you know) have probably been in the "no baby" situation for long enough that you and others are beginning to wonder.

You probably try to keep it from being obvious, but there are probably some telltale signs.

For whatever reason, up till now you have chosen not to tell of your infertility. At first the primary reason was that this was a temporary issue, one that would go away, so why tell anyone? If you haven't been infertile long, this may be the best course of action. Many couples have infertility problems for a short while, and the baby arrives after only a moderate delay.

But after a while, the reasons begin to change. Maybe you are not talking about it because you are afraid that people will feel sorry for you. Maybe you just don't want to hear the cruel and sometimes inappropriate things people will say. Maybe talking about it makes it seem more real and overwhelming. Maybe you are a quiet sort of person who doesn't easily share intense personal feelings with others. Maybe you just feel it is none of their business. Amazingly enough, some people will even believe that you must have done something wrong if you can't get pregnant. Of course, you haven't done anything wrong. If life worked that way, child abusers would never have children. You might not wish to share your infertility because you're afraid that people will try to make you feel guilty and broken.

Whatever the reason, most people experiencing infertility do not want anyone to know they are having problems trying to conceive or to carry a child to term, thus making it a private burden.

If you are among those who choose not to tell, you may miss out on the realization that there are a lot of other people out there who are having the same problem. This is understandable because those others often are not talking either. As a result you and your spouse may feel you are all alone. It is possible to become trapped in a cycle of isolation and depression.

I am not advocating that you shout it out to the world or take out an ad in the *Wall Street Journal*. But there is comfort and healing in knowing how many others are having similar infertility problems. You learn that you are not alone.

For us, being able to discuss it with others has been helpful. Writing about it has been extremely painful; yet we feel it is something we must do, and that gives us a sense of worth as we deal with not having children.

We hope to end the silence so that there may be healing for you or a loved one. We hope the stigma of infertility can be erased because the people who suffer from infertility are not to blame. They did not ask for this pain. They did nothing wrong. Yet to be denied something as vital and inherent as life itself is very hard to deal with.

Even given the reasons not to share, we still feel that being able to talk with someone who can understand is helpful. Obviously, one of the best ways to share is to talk with someone who understands how you feel, someone who is also walking the path of infertility.

You may have heard of a group called RESOLVE. RESOLVE is the National Infertility Association consisting of people who have experienced infertility and who are dedicated to helping infertile people. Someone in a RESOLVE group near you can probably understand and relate to your feelings of being out of control and grieving for the family you want. We highly recommend seeking them out early in your infertility journey. Most infertility specialists have the local number of a RESOLVE Chapter. If you are not able to find a local chapter, the national association may be able to help you find someone local. Check out www.resolve.org on the Internet.

The Internet has enabled people to talk about their infertility in ways that combine both privacy and sharing. There are many people sharing their infertility issues with each other over the 'Net. To find them, we recommend using a search engine and typing in the word infertility, or you can visit us at www.infertilitysanguish.com. Now that people have become comfortable with computers, the ability to share with others on the web anonymously has become a major way to begin the process of understanding that many people are going through infertility, and to find someone who can care and share.

If you are interested in using the Internet, but don't have a computer, check out your public library. Most libraries have Internet access as a free service.

If these options do not appeal to you, we still recommend that you do your best to find a special friend or relative who can be a sounding board.

Keeping it all inside does work for some. But if you find that you have traveled the road of infertility for a while, you really need to have some help carrying the load. First and foremost in sharing that load should be your spouse, but we hope you've been doing that all along. If you haven't, please be sure to read the section in this book titled: "How Do We Keep Communicating?"

Notes

— Do We Keep Quiet or Tell the World? —

You Are Not Alone

Dearest Jill,

Your letter was a Godsend! We haven't corresponded for a long time, but when I wrote to you last month, I didn't expect to hear that you were in a situation similar to mine.

I don't know what prompted me to get back in touch with you, other than the fact that I have been feeling lonely and cut off lately. Remembering the fun times we had together in college and afterwards made me wish again for those long conversations we used to have.

I'm so tempted to call, but I always worry how much it costs to call Australia, and the fine art of letter writing is calming.

When I wrote my letter to you, I know I must have gone on and on about all the routine things that have been going on in our lives. I almost didn't mention that we've been trying to have children but hadn't succeeded. I remember agonizing over whether to write that part since I didn't want to sound like I was consumed with self-pity. But I felt I needed to mention why I was not sending gushing news of our new baby like a lot of our friends have done. That sounds terrible, does it not? It's hard to sound objective about not having children.

Anyway, I must admit that I was completely surprised by your response telling me that you had been experiencing the same difficulty; that you were also unable to have children (so far). I know that you said you haven't told anyone, even though you were beginning to get questions from friends and relatives. I understand why you don't want to answer them.

I'm glad that you felt safe telling me, since you know I won't tell anyone else.

I got tears in my eyes, too, when I read your letter, just as you did reading mine. Knowing that you feel alone, too, somehow makes me feel as if I'm not strange or weird because of the feelings I've been having. I have to admit I'm stunned (and honored!) that my letter allowed you to open up and discuss your fears and hopes with me, even though you haven't done it with anyone else.

And, yes, please! I definitely want to keep writing and talking about this. I'd love to discuss all the absurd-sounding treatments we have to go through in the pursuit of having children. And I'd love to have a heart-to-heart talk about adoption.

In thinking back, I'm glad I didn't resist the urge to speak about my inability to have children. I think we both would have been a lot lonelier.

But, I agree with you and understand your reluctance to share your infertility with others. I'd like to tell you about one big mistake I made in sharing this problem with a friend in the neighborhood. I truly think she is well-meaning, but it's amazing how insensitive she can be.

First off, even though I told her privately, it didn't take long for the entire neighborhood to know. Now when I go through an infertility treatment, they all want to know the details and ask when I'm supposed to start my period. I'd even get phone calls right around then to see if I was pregnant or if I'd started my period.

They'd say things like, "We're wishing you the best," and "We sure hope you're pregnant." I can tell they're just plain curious; they want to know all about it. They are invading my privacy, and I've given them an excuse to do so.

The real problem is that I'm very depressed when my period starts and I don't need to talk to a bunch of busybodies.

Realizing There's A Problem

When I revealed my infertility to them, I hoped they would let me come talk to them when I felt like talking. Instead, they pester me when I have no interest in talking about it. I get so frustrated whenever I go through a procedure because I have to tell all of them it didn't work again. I decided at one point to stop talking about it to them at all, but they didn't want to give up knowing what was happening.

I guess I'm telling you this story to agree with you that not everyone should know what is going on. You have a right to keep it private.

On the other hand, I am so grateful that you are available for me to write to. Also, I do have one friend, Katherine, who understands, and whom I have been able to share things with. She listens when I need her to, and she waits for me to talk to her when I need to talk.

Katherine makes me feel less alone. I wanted to tell you about her, because your letter sounded very lonely. If you aren't sharing your problem with anyone, please continue to share with me. And if you can find someone you trust, I think you'll find talking about it will help. Even though I made a mistake with the neighbor, sharing with Katherine has helped me immensely.

You aren't alone. If you want to talk about it, I will read any letters you send. If you want to call, you can even call collect. I care. I'm willing to listen.

We're both suffering through this. I guess if we have to suffer, we can suffer together. And when it's all done, and we both have babies, I will arrange for a vacation to Australia to celebrate.

Love forever,
Even with the time and distance we're apart,
Alia

Notes

— Have We Done Something Wrong? —

The Sin of Infertility

You've accepted you have an infertility problem. Now you need to stop blaming yourself, or feeling guilty about why this is happening to you, or wonder why God has done this to you, or accept implied blame from others.

You need to treat yourself nicely, because unfortunately our society does expect you to blame yourself, because they assume you have done something wrong.

Blame from Society

Historically, infertility reaps very little pity, but quite a lot of blame. The woman was almost always the one blamed; she was the one who visibly didn't have children. Words like "barren" were spat out in disgust at women who could not fulfill the "biblical tradition" of being fruitful and multiplying.

As society evolved, the need for children was paramount. They were needed for farming. They were needed in quantity to ensure survival. They were needed to carry on the family traditions and defend the family lands. Not being able to have children was considered almost a sin; certainly not a medical condition that would be treated or accepted with compassion.

Women who couldn't bear children were often considered useless. England's King Henry VIII went through a total of six wives and a newly established religion trying to a produce a vigorous male heir. Certainly, the fact that he tired of his wives and often dallied with a new interest had something to do with it. But he often used the excuse of not having a vigorous male heir as a way to put them aside. Even today, with the knowledge of some of Henry's ulterior motives, some still validate Henry, seeing the need for the six wives based on the assumption that he needed male heirs to preserve the kingdom.

Women who cannot bear children are still often perceived negatively. Men who are not able to impregnate their wives are considered to shoot blanks. With today's medical advances, we've managed to extend the blame to both sexes. Society feels someone must be at fault when it comes to a lack of conception. Society and its citizens have trouble separating an undesired medical condition from a deliberate act.

Even in casual conversation, the issue can arise. The simple question, "Do you have children?" can bring up the specter of blame. In this case, the blame is often more general — it is the societal blame of not being normal, of not following the accepted path of life. It is the same blame as that of not being married by a certain age, of not having a checking account, of not being what you are expected to be based on your family background, your education and so on.

Many of us grow up hearing "God will get you for that" or "If you are bad you'll pay for it someday." Now all of a sudden what you consider a basic right is denied. "What did you do wrong?" people say. "You're overweight. You've been working too hard and the stress is causing you problems. Just take it easy. You shouldn't have refinished all that antique furniture; it is working with all of those chemicals that caused the problem. Why did you wear such tight clothes? Why did you wait so long to try to have children? You shouldn't have taken hot baths, or worn tight underwear." And on and on and on it goes.

Blame from Yourself

With all of this blame passed on to you by others, it is almost impossible not to buy into it yourself. As a result, you may begin to tell yourself you've sinned or are guilty.

You wanted to have children. You expected to have children. Now, all of a sudden, you can't. Your body is even telling you that you must. You crave babies. You get emotional thinking about babies. You feel your biological clock running.

Not surprisingly, you begin to go through a litany of blame. "Why do I have to be childless? Why am I the one to be broken? Have I done something in my past that is preventing me from having children? Is it the birth control that I used before I was ready to have children that is causing the problem? Did we wait too long? Are there reasons God is not blessing us? Are we being punished? If so, by whom and why? Can we change the situation? If we can, how? Why do others seem to be able to get pregnant so easily? Why are there so many pregnant women walking the shopping malls? Is it even possible for me to get pregnant? When will this nightmare end?"

After a while, this litany can begin to wear on your self-esteem. By accepting the blame, by beginning to believe there is something wrong with you versus your body, you may reach the point where you ask a more specific, blame-filled question like "Why are we the ones to be broken?" And when you ask this question, you no longer mean it in a physical sense, but in a sense of sin or guilt or blame.

Once you have started down this rocky road of blame, it becomes easy to blame others as well as yourself in order for you to get through the day. Maybe you'll begin to blame your spouse.

Maybe you'll begin to blame God. Many of those we've talked with, even those who would not call themselves religious, begin to wonder what sin they must have committed in order for this grief to have entered their lives. Many become very angry with God, saying it is God's fault.

Separation from Society

Have you started to see the vicious circle? Do you see that the acceptance of societal blame is a road to ruin? In blaming yourself, you begin to separate yourself from the society that blames you, as a way to live with yourself.

When this happens, we begin to avoid people who seem to be able to easily get pregnant, partially because we've bought into self-blame. Their pregnancy emphasizes the fact that we as infertile people must be broken. We don't fit anymore. We're not normal. Our friends with children have different interests. We want to have the same interests, but we feel left out. Having so far been denied one of the typical stages of life, the stage of parenthood, we have difficulty with our self-esteem.

We begin to snipe at others. We feel personally affronted when someone makes an unthinking but innocent statement like "It is too bad you have been unable to have children. You would make such good parents." We no longer quietly say "Thank you." Instead, we want to respond with bitter statements like:

- Yeah, I know!
- Do you have a crystal ball or are you naturally this astute?
- So what is keeping God from realizing that fact?
- Sincere thanks for understanding, but don't you wonder what terrible secret is causing this?

Feeling full of guilt and separated from others, we begin to go to any lengths to have children. But now it is in an attempt to be *normal*, not for the joy of children themselves.

Realizing There's A Problem

Separation from Yourself

As part of this vicious circle, having children becomes the paramount mission in your life. Sometimes even an obsession. Nothing else matters anymore. Your entire life becomes wrapped up in the cyclical events of procreation, and the blame is reinforced each time you are casually asked by someone, "How many children do you have? When do you plan to have some?"

Your day-to-day life becomes a blur. You go through the motions, but you have managed to separate yourself from your own life. Only the goal of having children remains.

Breaking the Vicious Circle

If you have arrived at this point, you need to tell yourself that infertility just *IS*, and do the best you can. Infertility should be looked at as more like a disease or a disability, not as sin or guilt.

When infertility is diagnosed, blame should never become part of future discussions, with others or with yourself. Infertility just *IS* and blame, guilt, remorse, etc., etc., etc., will never change the past. The present and the future are where *you* are. You need to accept that you are currently infertile. You need to decide on a constructive path to follow.

To break the cycle of blame, you probably need to continue to try to have children, but you need to make it *one* major important item in your life instead of the *only* important item in your life. You need to ensure that infertility does not consume you entirely.

You are important in other ways.

You have to continue with your life, whether you seek infertility treatment, decide to adopt, or accept being childfree. All of us are created equally, although differently from one another. We still have merit even if we are infertile. We have value. We count. We may not fit society's fairy-tale mold of the perfect people. But that is okay. We have a lot to contribute to society; even if what we contribute is not a child.

In writing this, we realize a lot of this is "do as we say, not as we did." Sometimes we wish that we could have some of the years back to redo them. Did we obsess? Yes, some. Did we blame ourselves? More than we'd like to admit. And, yes, some of those years seem like a blur. In hindsight, we wish we'd tried as hard to have children as we did, but it would have been nice had we not dwelled on it as much.

We would like to have been more accepting of ourselves. We would like to have been more forgiving of what we perceived to be our faults. We would like to have been able to more easily dismiss the comments of others, realizing that they probably didn't know how they were affecting us.

Had we done so, we would have had more time for the business of living, without shedding one iota of the time we took trying to have children.

Having children is a meaningful and worthwhile dream to pursue. Continue to walk that path of trying to have them, but in doing so, don't buy into the sin and guilt that may be placed upon you by society or by yourself.

We believe having children is a goal worth reaching for. But, so are your other dreams.

— Have We Done Something Wrong? —

Children Are Required

I wasn't surprised when our minister called. But I'll admit I was surprised by the directness of the questions he asked of Scott and me.

My church friends and minister had been wondering why we did not have children. At first, they were afraid to ask. I guess they thought we might reject their concern. Our church is full of family-type people. In fact, we chose our church because we wanted a large family.

When Scott and I married we wanted to finish college before we started our family, so we used birth control for a while. That didn't change the fact that we wanted a large family. Both of us come from families with many children, and we are encouraged by our faith to have a large family.

After finishing school, Scott got a good job. One day he came home from work full of excitement and said in a loud voice, "Julie! What do you think of being a mother to our children? What do you think about starting our family?"

We both burst out laughing with excitement and joy to think that at last we could begin the long-awaited family we had been postponing. We spent hours talking about the children we wanted and some of the names we liked. It was almost as if they were already born to us.

I had already seen a gynecologist for a routine checkup and he had said we should try to start our family soon if we did not want to have any difficulty. I was, after all, twenty-five years old. The doctor said not to worry; sometimes it takes up to a year to conceive.

I remember being frustrated when I was not pregnant by the fourth month and trying to tell myself that things really were okay. It was just taking a while like the doctor said it might. And my job did keep me busy, so I wasn't really worried. But when it had been ten months and I still was not pregnant, we did begin to worry.

We didn't mention to our friends that we were trying to have children. That would be admitting to having sex. So we just bottled up our feelings about how long it was taking to conceive. We did not even talk to each other about it. I guess we were just hoping that next month we would get pregnant.

It was about this time that our minister felt he needed to counsel us to begin to have children. After all, it was our privilege and responsibility to produce the next generation. Don't get me wrong; this man is a wonderful person. He was only echoing what we know to be our church's position on the bonding of husband and wife in marriage.

After the meeting with our minister, we became fearful that we might not be able to have children. What if we were barren? Were we less in God's eyes if we were barren? Weren't children a blessing from the Lord? Didn't he give them to us for caring and loving and educating? Were we not worthy of children?

This began a time of soul-searching. We wondered why we were broken. We questioned whether we had sinned by waiting to have children until we finished our education. Were we being punished for waiting or maybe for using birth control? As the months went by, we felt more and more guilty. What had we done wrong to deserve this lack of children? Why did our bodies not work the way they were supposed to?

Finally, after trying for a year and a half, we went to our minister to talk with him about our dilemma. We felt we could ask him our questions about what we must have done to deserve this treatment from God. He admitted that he had wondered if we were having trouble getting pregnant, but did not want to mention it in his first talk with us.

He told us that a lot of young couples had problems having children and gave us statistics on how often conception difficulties occurred. Often, couples had to go through medical treatment to have children, he added. I felt relieved when he assured us that God is a loving God and that God did not deliberately single us out to be barren. Our minister encouraged us to go to a specialist for some testing. He even had a doctor to recommend.

I'm glad our minister did not say words that would keep us feeling guilty and sinful. I am also glad he helped us to see that we were feeling out of control. Sometimes we don't know what is in store for us, but he counseled us to pray and ask God for guidance. We needed to keep from rejecting God in our bitterness. We needed to trust in God for help.

After that, I talked with other women whom I met at the doctor's office where I was receiving infertility treatments. Some of them had gone through some of the same guilt and sinful feelings. They were mad at God and blamed him for their lack of children. I realized I was not alone in blaming God for my pain and sorrow. I also was not alone in thinking I had done something wrong and God was punishing me.

Happily, I can say that we finally did receive our blessing from God. She is every bit as precious as we dreamed. Our daughter helps us see that God loves and cares for us.

Notes

— Why Doesn't My Family Understand? —

Related Opinions

How many times have your parents or in-laws asked where their grandchildren are? If you've been on the road of infertility for a while, that topic has been brought up at least once. Even if they have other grandchildren, they want to know when *you* will be having children.

Why do they ask? For the same reason they wonder if they can afford to send you to college. For the same reason they wonder whom you will marry. For the same reason they wonder how your job is going. Having kids is one of the steps to growing up in our society. Until you've accomplished that task, you haven't fully moved into the grown-up world, and your parents are concerned.

That doesn't mean that their concern would stop once you did have kids. Then they'd wonder how well you are raising them. But the point is that your parents want to see you succeed in taking the next normal step in your life. And that next step affects them. They often want grandchildren because that's the next normal step in their lives.

If you have been on the road of infertility long enough, your brothers, sisters, and even your third cousin may be asking about your missing children.

For a while, you've smiled (through gritted teeth) and said, "Oh, we're still thinking about it" or "We'll let you know when it happens" and hoped that would quiet the questions. If you're lucky, your relatives have considered that to be enough, and have let you go about your business in our children-producing world.

After a while, especially if you haven't shared your reasons for not having children, the persistent questions combined with your attempts at childbearing can wear you down. At this point, you usually have two choices. You can either continue to keep your infertility journey private, or you can share the information with some of your family.

This is not an easy decision. Unlike telling a close friend who would understand, you can't pick and choose your relatives. You may have parents who would be extremely helpful once they knew your plight. Conversely, you might have relatives who would look at you in disbelief, and make comments that would make the situation even worse.

When it comes to telling family, you have to make a personal value judgment. All families have blessings and problems. Some families argue over money, some experience sibling rivalry, some are estranged and some get along quite well. Infertility adds one more item to the family equation. You need to decide if sharing this information will generate good or bad will.

Of course, the final reality is that either decision will end up being a mixed blessing. If you keep the whole situation private, the questions will probably continue or incorrect assumptions will be made. If you share, you may achieve some level of understanding and sympathy, but may open up new areas of misunderstanding since they will expect you to provide progress reports on your status to conceive.

The largest area of potential conflict occurs because your relatives will most likely want to "help" you solve your problem. Your parents have helped you before, so why shouldn't they help you now? It's natural, right?

Other than the same help offered by friends, that of commiseration, understanding, and love, almost anything offered by your relatives will be inappropriate. And it will be very hard for you to tell them that. They want to help. A lot of times they don't understand that what you are going through is something they cannot help you with. It is a wise parent who does understand your need to solve this yourself.

Your hope is that they will provide the support necessary for you to endure the infertility journey. Your fear is that they will tell you what to do to fix things.

- They might recommend certain medical tests for you to take, all the while not understanding what you've already gone through, or what is appropriate. They might even set up a doctor's appointment for you.
- If you have a period or miscarry, they could say inappropriate things like "It's not a big deal" or "You weren't really very pregnant."
- If you're the man, your parents might take you aside and say, "At least it's not as important to the man to have kids. You still have your career." They are trying to make you feel better, but they don't understand that you might want children as much as your wife.
- Eventually, they might tell you how adopting would solve all your problems, even before you've gotten to that point. In the worst case, they would continue to find "solutions" to your problems without understanding the problems you face.

If you have an extremely understanding family only some or none of these things might occur. It can make your infertility journey an easier one.

Since you must make this decision on how much to share of your infertility crisis with your family; we certainly hope that you can reach a positive conclusion in this matter.

Notes

— Why Doesn't My Family Understand? —

A Test of Wills

How does a man tell his parents that he can't have children? It is an awkward situation at best. I guess eventually they suspect it, but for the first few years it is not an easy subject to broach, even when you have a good relationship with them.

In our case, both sets of our parents are fixated on their grandchildren. That's not a bad thing, except that we don't have any for them to be fixated on.

Last year, we were visiting my parents, and with everyone present, they began joking about having grandchildren. They said that if only Steve and Donna would take a little trip upstairs they could bring you some cousins. As if we had not already thought of that very idea. Imagine that! My parents raising a child so stupid that he did not know what caused pregnancy.

Well, it felt that way at least. When we did not take the hint, everyone laughed, I guess to relieve the tension of a crude joke. But the funny part was when little Jim asked Grandpa why our children would come from upstairs, when all the babies in his family came from the hospital. My father just laughed it off and the conversation went on, with everyone oblivious to how much pain we were in. Whoever said there was a good reason to have a poker face? Maybe if our pain showed, they would be more in tune with how we felt.

✧ ✧ ✧

Early this fall, something similar happened when we were visiting Donna's parents. They informed us that for the coming holiday season they were still going to get Christmas presents for the grandchildren, but they would not have enough money to buy gifts for their grown children. But, of course, that would be okay, they added, since the grown children didn't need presents. After all, Christmas was for children.

Should we have told them we felt left out? Should we have told them that we have been trying for nearly three years and had been diagnosed as being infertile with little hope of having children?

We didn't say anything. Instead we cried. It really hurt. It wasn't the money. It was the very thought of being left out of Christmas by one's parents and having to enjoy our nieces and nephews getting presents when we didn't have children who could participate. It seemed to be a sign of failure that we could not produce like we should.

That night Donna and I discussed if her parents were being cruel or just dense. The next day we tried to tell Donna's parents the problems we were having in conceiving a child. I thought I was stubborn! They had fixed in their minds that since all of their children were out of the nest, on their own, and at least moderately successful, we did not need presents. When we were successful in having children, they would get presents. Until then, what was the difference? We couldn't get them to understand that we felt left out.

When Donna realized it was futile, she blurted out, "That's fine, if that is the way you want to be, we have two cats and they would enjoy some fresh catnip and liver treats for their birthdays." She even named the days of their birth. Unfortunately, instead of conveying the point, this comment got Donna's mom angry and she declared she was not going to buy toys for cats when she had precious grandbabies to buy for. I was proud of Donna. She did not break down and cry. She would later, I knew, but she took it calmly and realized she was not going to be able to get her parents to understand. Somehow they thought it was all because we did not want to have children yet, even though we told them differently.

Maybe that is the problem with infertility today. We are so concerned with waiting to start our family until we can afford to that we convey the image that we will try when we feel it is time. People assume we are still waiting instead of having problems conceiving.

✧ ✧ ✧

Realizing There's A Problem

The real shocker came yesterday. When my Dad had a mild heart attack last spring the doctor scared him into eating right and quitting smoking, but Mom scared him even more when she insisted they get a will made up. She was not going to let him die intestate and leave her with all the headaches that causes, especially given that they had a fairly sizable estate. As I was the oldest, I was named executor. I was not consulted about any of this, it was done and I was informed afterwards. I guess that's usual for parents who are self-sufficient.

At any rate, I got a call last week asking me if I could drive the three hours this weekend to look over some legal papers. Of course, Donna and I said sure.

I got the shock of my life when I read my parents' will. There were a lot of estate and trust complexities, but basically it stated that all their assets and moneys derived from the sale of property were to be divided in equal amounts among their grandchildren. There were no monetary provisions for any of their children.

Both of my parents looked at me expectantly and asked if they had done the right thing. The way the question was asked left no doubt that I was expected to congratulate them on how fair-minded they had been and how this would be wonderful, because now all of the grandkids would have the necessary money to go to college. We weren't being slighted, of course. Our children would be provided for as well.

I was speechless. Maybe we were being selfish, but Donna and I had spent all our savings on infertility treatments rather than on the children we wanted to have. We had hoped that in the future, truly hoping it would be very distant, that we might inherit some money that could be put aside for retirement. Now I was being asked to help settle my parents' estate and give the proceeds to my nieces and nephews and get punished for not having children. I sat there silently for so long the lawyer finally asked if I was okay.

To tell you the truth, I am not sure what I did next. I don't know if I ranted and raved, or if I walked out without saying a word. I was in shock. The pain of the last three years came crashing in on me. Again, as I had many times before, I thought of the time in football when I was thrown to the ground. Was that the time my testicle got torqued, causing damage and resulting in a non-existent sperm count, or was it the time I fell in basketball and three others fell on top of me? Or was it both? I was sure my problem was caused by a sport injury. If it had not been for that injury we would not be going through this. Regardless, all I really know is that I was not coherent enough to express to my parents what I was really feeling especially in front of a lawyer writing a will.

Donna was there for me. She drove home. She held me and let me cry. She let me talk, and when I was finished for a while she held me some more.

This morning, I found the courage to call my parents and ask them if we could talk. I apologized for walking out on the conference with the lawyer and told them I wanted to explain things to them. We're driving back now. I want to talk to them in person. The next few hours are going to be rough.

— Why Does the Man Care? —

Life Goes On

There is a definite perception that the group that walks the road of infertility is made up primarily, if not exclusively, of women.

The basic assumption is that the woman is the one who has problems with infertility. The primary interest a man has is to help satisfy his wife's need to have children. Society often perceives that the man really does not care if he has children or not. A man has other interests. His career will carry him through any minor discomforts or anguishes he might feel during the infertility process. The concept that a man could mourn a lack of children is foreign to most people who haven't dealt with the problem themselves.

Even among those experiencing infertility directly, each member of a couple may have distinctly different views of what the other is feeling.

Her: "I know my husband cares, but whenever I want to discuss trying harder to have kids, he always brings up something he has to do for work. But I can't ignore it like he can. We're doing artificial insemination, so all he has to do is provide a sperm sample once or twice a month, and then he can forget the whole thing. I have to be part of the process every day. I have to watch my body calendar, my temperature charts, and I have to make sure I take my medicine in the proper dosage at the right time. With all that, I can't ignore it; I can't use work as an excuse to forget about infertility."

Him: "I don't know what she wants me to do. I always make sure I do whatever she asks me to do. She gets crazy from the medicine, and I do my best to be there for her. When her period starts, I'm there for her when she is angry or cries, or whatever. I don't know what more there is to talk about. We've talked about it too much as it is. I have to earn a living. I have to make sure we can afford the baby if it ever shows up.

Do I want a kid? Of course, I do. Do you think I'd go through all this grief if I didn't?"

Historically, our society has decided that having and caring for kids is the woman's job and responsibility. So naturally, solving the infertility problem has also fallen into the woman's realm of responsibility and for that reason, infertility is not considered something the man has to solve.

No wonder society thinks that a man shouldn't be concerned when he hasn't had children. Society considers a man more important based on what he can accomplish in a business, economic, or provider sense. This remains true even considering the long-term trend of women entering the workplace, and of men spending more time with their children. The views of society are shaped over centuries and change very slowly.

So, Does the Man Care?

Most men have always cared. They may not emotionally show it. They may not know how to express it, and they may not want people to know they care. But, yes, men do care.

Men do not care in the same way that women do. This difference, a basic sexual one, is a major reason that couples wonder why the other one doesn't understand.

Before we go further, let's set some ground rules. Generalizations are about to be made. Whenever one makes statements about groups, especially groups as pervasive as about half of the world's population, there will be exceptions. If the statement is made, "Men don't eat quiche," that may be true for most men, or many men, but there will be many people who can say, "I eat quiche" or "my husband eats quiche." Nonetheless, generalizations can be helpful as long as one realizes there are always exceptions.

Women, by nature, are nurturers. Men are not nurturers. Thus, women want babies, who require nurturing. Men want children. Men would probably be quite satisfied if women gave birth to three-year-olds who were potty trained as opposed to infants.

If asked, a man could probably not tell you exactly why he wants children (not babies). However, through numerous interviews, we have found three major reasons why men want children, as opposed to the default reason of wanting to please their spouse. These reasons are often distinctly different from why women want children. The three reasons are:

1. A desire for immortality;
2. A desire to mentor and teach; to pass on what they have learned in life;
3. A desire to return to innocence; to revisit childhood themselves.

Although other reasons are occasionally mentioned, they can almost always be fit into these three categories. And yes, even less occasionally, reasons like nurturing do come up to spoil the generality.

A Desire for Immortality

Men want to be immortal. Unfortunately, our bodies don't allow that. Having children to continue life is the only method open to men that allows them immortality. This desire is seen most clearly in regal dynasties where having a child (almost always male) was the requirement in order to say "The King Is Dead, Long Live the King!" The statement would signify the king's immortality through the existence of his child.

Depending on the strength of this desire, genetic continuity may be important to the man. He may not want to adopt because having a biological child is the only thing that fulfills this desire. For other men, adopting may be fine, because the immortality is achieved by passing on that which the man has learned in life to the child.

My most interesting take on immortality came from my doctor. He was intrigued about our infertility book and revealed that he had been unable to have children himself. He had discovered that inability at age sixteen, when he had observed his own sperm sample under the microscope. During his marriage, he had considered adoption, but as the marriage had difficulty, he abandoned the idea. He said that he didn't mind that he had never had children, but he admitted that he occasionally had to come to grips with it. In particular, he had trouble with what he called continuity.

He asked me when life began. Thinking he was bringing up an abortion topic, I replied, carefully, that it depended on what one believed. Some thought it was at conception, others at birth, and some societies even after birth. He pressed me, and I said that technically, life probably began at conception.

He replied, "You're wrong; totally wrong." He was extremely certain, and continued: "Life began millions of years ago."

"Life doesn't begin anymore, it continues. Having a child is a way to continue life into the future — it's a way to give oneself a form of immortality."

That was what he had to come to grips with; the fact that he couldn't continue life. His best coping mechanism was his brother's children. If he looked at his genetic background, he could look back to his parents, who continued life through him and his brother. In a sense, therefore, his brother continued my doctor's life by having children that were genetically tied to him.

For men who want their life to continue after they are gone, children are the only real way to do this. Men can look to their accomplishments and hope that they are forever remembered, but there are very few individuals who can hope for such recognition. Usually, a man is happy if he has children who carry on after him, even more so if directly tied to his own life and learning. Have you ever seen a man more proud than when he has a sign painter erect a new sign proclaiming "Smith & Sons" (or, today, "Smith & Daughter")?

A Desire to Mentor and Teach

This reason for wanting children is related to immortality in that a man wants to pass on the valuable things he has learned in life. When this desire is extremely strong, it may not matter if the child a man raises is biologically his.

We've all seen athletic men who buy ball gloves for their kids before they are out of diapers. "He'll be a chip off the old block!" they'll proclaim. Similarly, intellectual men are proud of their children's academic accomplishments. Men may also be proud when the child excels in ways different than the way they themselves excelled. In this case, a man fulfills his desire to revisit his own childhood through the child by vicariously excelling in this new area.

Historically, a man would pass on his trade to his son. This fulfilled immortality and teaching. Today, a man is proud to pass on his values and what he has learned. To have an adult child who reacts to society in a way similar to the way the father would react is a proud accomplishment.

This desire isn't limited to the major events. Simply teaching how to tie a shoe, to swim, to fly a kite — all of these fulfill the need to teach and to revisit childhood. The reasons for raising children blur, but they all tend to focus on moving the needs, values, wants, and thoughts of the father to the child.

In this way, the father is a success. His life is not transient. He lives forever through his children.

A Desire to Return to Innocence

We all grow up faster than we want to. Taking on responsibilities in the world removes much of our ability to just have fun. As adults, we have to seek out acceptable ways to abdicate our roles. There aren't too many. Vacations are acceptable, although short-term. Watching TV or reading a book is an acceptable escape from responsibility, but isn't as active as it could be.

Having a child – now that's a major way to escape. It's perfectly acceptable to relive your childhood through your child. You can go to Little League ball games, play catch, or enjoy Disney World without guilt. You can watch your child in school plays and remember how much you wanted to be an actor. You make time to go swimming and to have fun, because the kids need to go. You might not have done it if it were only for yourself.

And kids are the perfect acceptable excuse. "I can't work late because I have to pick up the kids and take them to the ballgame" is a society-approved statement, whereas "I want to go to the ballgame" is not.

The Man Just Cares Differently

Men want children. Women want babies. These are not incompatible desires, since babies become children very quickly. A man may even be happy to help diaper and nurture a baby, because it happens to fit in with his own individual nurturing abilities.

Unfortunately, because of the nature of men and the perceptions of society, a man may not make clear how much he does care. It appears as if he is only trying to meet his wife's needs to have children, not his own. In reality, a man has to live through his own private pain in not having children. Often, because he is not comfortable sharing his feelings, even his wife does not understand what he is going through.

Living forever is a tough proposition. Passing on what one has accomplished is not taken lightly. Continuing to be a child is a hard thing to achieve. None of these is discussed easily.

— Why Does the Man Care? —

The Story of G'Nor

The buds on the branches were opening. The long cold was ending; it was time once again to move forward. G'Nor took one of the buds and opened it carefully. Its intricacy always amazed him.

G'Nor called to his men. "It is time. Prepare for battle!"

G'Nor was an impressive sight. The tallest of all his tribe, he was the only one remaining with flaming red hair. Barely into his twentieth season, he had already commanded his people for almost four years. As his people spread across the lands, their tribe slowly grew; those they conquered who wished to join them in their grand travels replaced those lost in battle.

G'Nor looked from the hill down upon his people. He was proud of their activity. He was proud of what he had accomplished. Had it not been G'Nor who had figured out how to make their spears sharper and harder? Had it not been G'Nor who had figured out how to surround his enemies and always defeat them?

And, had it not been G'Nor who knew that it was best *not* to kill his enemies, but instead to recruit them to join? How else could he have put together the largest group in the area? How else could he be both feared and loved by those around him?

G'Nor walked through the camp, suggesting and helping as he went along. When he reached his private tent, the three women he had chosen to be his own awaited him eagerly. They offered him the best tidbits of the boar they had just prepared. But he wasn't interested in the boar. The new buds had intrigued him; he wanted to create some new life of his own.

✧ ✧ ✧

Five more seasons had passed. G'Nor's tribe was larger than ever; his fame had spread over the entire region. Rarely did he have to fight as they traveled. Instead, tribute was often given as G'Nor would promise protection to those who would submit. In trade for a village's offerings, G'Nor would often leave some of his fighting men who were tired of traveling as protectors.

But G'Nor was not happy. He was alone among his people. His flaming red hair set him apart; his height made him feel different. His two brothers were long dead; there was no one left from the small ragtag group from whence he had started his rise to greatness.

And none of the five women who were his alone had granted him an heir. He sighed, continuing to meditate alone in the grassy field with the heat of the summer sun beating down upon him. He was trying to understand the thoughts of the birds of the air, to sense the grass as it waved in the wind.

How he wanted to share these meditations. Most men feared him even as they admired him; even his trusted commanders were more entranced with conquering and fighting than he was. He knew that he had to fight to be strong; that was part of life. Nature itself showed him that; the strong survived; the weak died.

But he also saw the ants. No one watched them as he did. They cooperated; they thrived. Even when trampled by those stronger than them, they always came back, because they had an inner strength from their numbers and their unity.

He observed nature and how it worked. He applied that to his life. His learning had made him strong. When he tried to share that with others, they didn't understand. But a son! A son would give him back the joy that his life once had. With a son, he could see again for the first time. He could share these things of nature. He could share what he had learned. He could pass it on so it would not be forgotten.

Realizing There's A Problem

✧ ✧ ✧

Another fall had come and gone. It was fall again. G'Nor had stopped advancing his armies. He had decided that enough land had been taken; more of his people were now farmers instead of fighters. To move on now would only be to promote and advocate killing and destroying for its own sake; he had established a stable environment where his people could prosper.

But G'Nor's commanders were displeased. They cajoled him, they enticed him. "What do you mean, we have conquered enough? There are always more lands to be taken. We are strong now, but we can be stronger! You've said yourself that if we do not grow, we begin to die."

G'Nor looked up from the two boys he was trying to teach toward his commanders. He was trying to show them about the cycles of nature in the changing of the leaves. But they had already lost interest; the eight-year-olds were more fascinated by the entreaties of their fathers than they were by colored leaves.

"There are ways to grow other than by conquering," said G'Nor. He stood up and towered over his two commanders. The boys ran to their fathers as if to protect them from G'Nor's wrath. But G'Nor simply sighed and began to walk away.

"You've become weak!" shouted one, emboldened by G'Nor's attitude. "Has your failure as a man in bed made you a failure in battle as well? If you must take our sons, at least teach them something important like how to win a war! You taught us well, that is why we thought you could teach them." Sensing G'Nor's anger, he continued, "You are the great G'Nor! Continue to show us what made you great."

"You only see the beginning!" rebuked G'Nor. "At first, warriors enable us to grow and prosper. But once our community has reached a certain size, we must protect our people as well. We must stabilize what we have before we can expand further, otherwise we will be vulnerable." G'Nor began to say more but realized he was not making sense to any of the four standing before him.

He looked at the two boys standing in front of their fathers. They admired the great G'Nor, and wanted to learn from him. But they wanted to learn to fight; they wanted to learn how to be like their fathers. G'Nor placed his hands in front of him as if to put them on the shoulders of his own eight-year-old son, but instead finished by placing them upon his hips.

His son would understand. His son would learn how to fight and how to win, but would also learn what would come after. His son would ensure that what G'Nor had built would continue.

❖ ❖ ❖

During the winter, the arguments ceased, since the commanders' and G'Nor's wishes to not wage war matched, albeit for different reasons. And, to G'Nor's joy, one of his five women showed that she was to have a child. There was much talk and much jealousy among the other women, but finally G'Nor would have an heir.

❖ ❖ ❖

When spring arrived, G'Nor made two major decisions. First, he sent his commanders to the outer regions of the community to patrol, and if need be, to fight any potential invaders. For the first time, he did not accompany them. He was older now, almost twenty-eight, and he was sensing his own mortality. Although the farming men in his community lived longer, a warrior was old in his thirties. He wanted to live long enough to raise his son, to ensure that he could once again be young himself through his child, and to make sure that what he had created would continue.

Second, he had decided to be selfish for once and to declare a festival for the birth of his child. As the midwives worked, the preparations for festival were being made. The situation was stressful; everyone knew that something might go wrong, although the pregnancy appeared uneventful.

Realizing There's A Problem

G'Nor stood outside the birthing tent. He paced back and forth expectantly. When he heard a gasp from one of the women inside the tent, he immediately rushed in. One of the midwives tried to block his way. He heard the healthy wail of a baby. Why were they trying to stop him from entering? It was obvious that the birth had gone well. He brushed her aside and stepped forward. He stood regally, his flaming red hair reflecting from the torches. The blond-haired mother lay there, trembling, as one of the midwives cautiously put the healthy black-haired baby boy in her arms. The midwife wouldn't look into G'Nor's eyes.

"Who is the father!" bellowed G'Nor.

"Forgive me, my lord!" said the mother. "I truly thought the baby was yours! Would I have risked your wrath had I thought otherwise? I lay with another only twice, and it did not seem as if it were the right time for him to be the father."

"You have broken our laws, you have broken your oath, and you have broken my heart!" G'Nor shouted this through clenched teeth. "Who is the father?"

"Have mercy, my lord! He is but a simple farmer who caught my fancy. Neither of us intended to insult your greatness!"

One of the midwives whispered to G'Nor. "Kill the baby now. We can say it was stillborn. All of us are loyal to you; even she is, in her own way. You have done so much good. A bastard like this can only hurt how people feel about you."

"No. Bring all three of them to the festival area. Now! She looks healthy enough, even given the birth."

✧ ✧ ✧

It was hot. The sun beat down upon the screaming crowd. G'Nor stood tall and majestic among the smaller people around him. His red hair set him apart. He was alone among many.

The black-haired farmer was abased before G'Nor, mumbling about G'Nor's greatness. The blonde-haired mother held the baby, but in a way that suggested she didn't know whether to hold it tightly or hurl it from her. She and the baby were bawling.

G'Nor's voice rose above them all. The crowd was silent. "Our laws decree that a woman is bonded to a man. That no woman should leave her man without his consent; and that no man should take a woman bonded to another. The penalty for such transgressions is death by stoning."

The hot sun made G'Nor squint. He brushed his hand across his forehead. As his hand came down, he imagined that he grasped the shoulder of his ten-year-old son. "See the crowd," he whispered to his son. "All they know is fighting, killing, and revenge. They want me to issue the command to kill. But I have learned that there is more to life than killing. Justice must be mingled with mercy."

"I am a warrior. I learned how to destroy the weak so that the strong would flourish. You must learn how to deal with our community, so that they may be even stronger, or all of my hopes and dreams will die with me."

"We have a chance here to make a statement, one of cooperation rather than one of revenge. Do you understand, my son?"

A cloud crossed the path of the sun. The noise of the crowd interrupted the silence within G'Nor. He looked at his hand; all it grasped was the hilt of his sword. He saw the fervor of the crowd around him. They only understood him as a warrior, a person of strength, a person of power. No one understood what else he knew.

"Kill them!" shouted G'Nor.

Stones began to fly, but G'Nor himself walked quickly away. He had taken the stance he knew his people expected, but he no longer cared. He knew now that he would always be alone. He would never have anyone to whom he could pass on his thoughts, his cares, his desires, or his hopes. He walked into his tent; he dismissed his wives even as they tried to comfort him.

❖ ❖ ❖

G'Nor rejoined his armies. His commanders welcomed him back. He was his old self again! The next spring, G'Nor expanded his region more than he ever had before. He simply smiled wanly when he was given the news that some of the regions that they had acquired years ago were under attack by other forces nearby. He simply said that they had gained more than they lost. His commanders approved, since they could continue to advance. They didn't understand his cryptic comment, "The flower that lives the shortest often has the most beauty."

On the eve of his thirty-second birthday, G'Nor led an attack on a village that wouldn't yield to his entreaties to surrender. He was impaled on a spike by a farmer defending his land. The village was conquered, but during the next few weeks, G'Nor's deep shoulder wound festered and infected his body. G'Nor died soon thereafter.

G'Nor's death heralded the quick breakup of his realm. It was too large; there was no cohesive force to keep it together. Within a few short seasons, small bands of warriors roamed again; the peace of G'Nor's realm was quickly lost. It was not long before all was as it had been before.

G'Nor was no more.

Notes

— How Do We Keep Communicating? —

Honesty, the Best Medicine

As you travel the road of infertility, it is much easier to travel with a companion than to travel alone. That companion may be a sympathetic friend or an understanding family member, but the best travel partner you can have would be an understanding and sympathetic spouse.

Unfortunately, the two individuals who make up a couple may not be fully communicating when dealing with infertility. You may be at different points along the infertility road. Thus, you may both be dealing with the problem, but separately.

Dealing with infertility within a partnership isn't any different than dealing with any major problem. Infertility is one of the "for worse" items in the marriage vows that you took. Your fertility is not something that either of you decided to sabotage. Even if your partner got a vasectomy or a tubal ligation during a previous marriage, it wasn't a slight against you.

Infertility is something that needs to be dealt with openly between a couple, and it becomes easier if you both realize that you are in fact in this as a couple. Unfortunately, rather than talking about the infertility, what often results is the passing of blame, guilt, grumpiness, nastiness, or simple avoidance. Any major crisis in a marriage is an opportunity to either pull together or to push apart.

If you take your anger out on your spouse, it will only hurt matters. You may think that because you are close to that person, they will still love you after you finish lashing out. But anger always takes its toll. It is also fruitless to bring in blame. Blame will ultimately undermine and destroy your relationship.

If infertility is causing a rift in your relationship, you may need to consult a lot more than this book. Are there other areas where you are pulling apart? If so, you might need to evaluate your marriage in general, and work on how to keep it together. If it is only infertility, that still can be enough to drive you apart. Look to the ways where you do get along. Try to apply the techniques that work for you in other areas to your infertility issues.

As stated earlier, we do not have the perfect solution. There are many days of our lives we wish we could have back again when we had arguments, misunderstandings, and just plain couldn't agree on what to do next.

We tried to remain close together. Our rule in communication was to hold nothing back. We tried not to falsely blame one another or spread guilt just to hurt. If there was resentment, we laid it on the table and talked about it. We also tried to praise each other as much as possible. It's amazing how much a simple "thank you" when dinner is cooked, the lawn is mowed, or a room is cleaned can help when you find yourself in an argument later on. Just knowing that your spouse does care can make you be less bitter when that inevitable "discussion" on infertility occurs.

So, based on our personal experiences, we come to the same conclusion as almost all of the psychology books: communicate. Unlike your friends, unlike your family, your partner is someone you have to deal with every day. You can choose to not discuss the issue, but in the long run, an issue not discussed becomes a wedge that can drive the two of you apart; until you find that you are living with a stranger.

Try to use infertility as a way to grow closer. Get closer to each other on the infertility road by discussing where each of you is in that journey. Do you both really want a baby? How much? What are you willing to do to end up with a child? How much infertility treatment would you consider?

You may find that you didn't even know where your partner really was about the entire issue. Use what you learn to better understand where the other is coming from. Develop ways to help one another through the days when you lose hope of ever having children. Decide together

Realizing There's A Problem

whom you will tell about what you are going through. Work toward always dealing with each issue together rather than separately.

We're not suggesting that this will be easy. If the two of you are of a like mind in handling infertility issues, it may not be hard to be successful in taking this journey together. But if you are at two different points in life on how to deal with infertility, you may find that you are traveling the road alone. However, if you do end up traveling alone, remember that the most desired way to leave the path of infertility is to have a child. If you decide it is okay to travel alone while experiencing infertility, make sure that you won't also be traveling alone if you succeed in having a baby.

Infertility is just one major issue you have to deal with as a couple. Do your best together; examine what it means if you continue to deal with it separately. You owe it to yourself and to your future child to be as successful as possible in communicating with your spouse.

Notes

— How Do We Keep Communicating? —

What's So Funny?

Connie says I don't ever take this infertility stuff seriously. She's on Pergonal and has emotional jags that range from giddiness to severe depression. I just sigh and say I'm trying to absorb her few good moods so they don't drain away.

I mean, you can allow yourself to be depressed or you can take situations as best as possible, right? I'd rather see the lighter side of things than be depressed. It helps me get through tough situations.

Connie, on the other hand, stays depressed almost constantly. What do you say to a woman who can come home from the shopping mall bawling her eyes out? "Were all the outfits you looked at polka-dotted or something?" I queried.

"I had to leave. There were **babies** there!" she said.

"Why? Were they all polka-dotted?"

She ignored me. "I shouldn't go to the mall during weekday work hours. All the mothers and their cute little babies were waiting there for me. As soon as I saw them, I had to leave. I just couldn't stay!"

"Why? Were they waiting to ambush you when you entered?" I imagined a bunch of three-year-olds with light sabers in military formation in the mall corridors. When Connie arrived, they would attack her with the buzz-buzz-buzz of their little toy swords. "Did the mothers have placards saying 'I have a baby and you don't'?"

Connie didn't think it was funny. I got cold pizza for dinner that night.

Later that week, we were headed to the big football game across state. On entering the rival city, we saw billboards everywhere proclaiming

"Baby Sale!" with a picture of a cute baby and the store name on it. Connie said the signs reminded her of the mall trip.

When we passed the store, I couldn't resist. I pulled into the parking lot and motioned Connie to come with me. She knows that gleam in my eye, so she didn't say anything. We entered the store and approached the counter. I got a sales clerk's attention and said loudly, "We'll take two!"

"Two what?" she said, sounding slightly irritated and bored.

"Two babies, of course." To my delight, Connie started giggling.

"The baby sale is for baby clothing." Obviously, she had no sense of humor. Or maybe it was the green and white rival colors we were wearing.

"All the signs say 'Baby Sale'! And, you know, I like the look of the cute baby on Highway 23. Is he still available? Price is no object! Or are you all out of the cute ones?"

The clerk just stared at me. Connie started laughing and pounded my shoulder. I shrugged, as if to assume that if the clerk were quiet, the store must be out of babies. "Maybe another store will still have some," I commiserated, as we turned to leave.

That put Connie in a much better mood for the ball game. The fact we were winning helped, too. So it was actually in a decent tone of voice when Connie reminded me that we needed to give her a Pergonal shot.

"Can it wait till after the game?" I asked. No, of course not, I said to myself.

We left our seats, but couldn't find a private area. We asked where the infirmary was, but couldn't locate it. Climbing a set of stairs, I noticed we were totally alone, so I said, "I've got this down pat. Drop your pants and I'll plug you right here."

Connie knows I can do it quickly, so she lowered her jeans and I gave her the shot. Wouldn't you know that a group of college frat boys dressed in yellow and blue started up the stairs right then?

Realizing There's A Problem

What else could I do? As Connie quickly hiked up her pants, I mooned them as well, to distract their attention. We rushed around the corner. I thought they'd follow us, but they didn't. Connie burst out, "Did you want a shot, too?"

"Just a shot of whiskey, please, my dear," I responded.

After winning the game, Connie insisted on driving home because she wanted me to read one of those medical infertility books. She says I don't pay enough attention to the process. Hey, I pay attention. She just doesn't think I do.

She must have been eyeing shopping malls, because on the way home, she said, "I still need a new outfit. Hmm, how many pairs of jeans do you have?"

I acted as if I was intently studying the medical texts. "Twenty-three pair;" I responded, as if to a pop quiz.

"No, no, no. I mean blue jeans."

"I really don't think any of my genes are blue. Blue balls, maybe."

"Cut it out. Anyway, that's chromosomes! See. You don't pay attention!"

Well, that one didn't work. The next day, I had to give my sperm sample so Connie could be inseminated. We went to the doctor's office together. The nurse gave me a sperm cup and asked me if I wanted *Playboy*, *Penthouse*, or *Hustler* when I went to the "little room."

"Actually, I'd like Connie, if that's ok with you ..." I smiled. So did Connie. This part was never easy. Everyone knows what you do in the "little room." But, hey, make the best of it.

This morning, Connie announced that her period had started. I was reading the paper, so I just set it aside, and put my arms up in the air. She came over and I hugged her and held her close while she cried.

I don't make jokes at a time like this.

Notes

Part 2
Trying to Get Pregnant

Seeking Help, Choosing a Doctor

    When it Takes More Than Two   79
    The Bookstore   87

Handling Drugs and Surgery

    Treatment: Blessing or Curse?   91
    Interruptions   95

Examining Alternative Pregnancies

    Breaking the Rules   103
    Beating the System   107

Considering Prayer

    Prayer: Can it Help?   111
    The Patience of John   113

78 Infertility's Anguish

Quote on page 101 is from the song
I Dreamed a Dream from *Les Miserables*
lyrics by Alain Boublil, Herbert Kretzmer, & Jean-Marc Natel
music by Claude-Michel Schönberg
Copyright 1986
Alain Boublil MusicLtd.

— Seeking Help, Choosing a Doctor —

When It Takes More than Two

As we mentioned earlier, you are *not* reading an authoritative book on medicines or medical doctors. If anything, pretend we're sitting in a lounge, taking a short break during our infertility journey, having a conversation about how that journey feels.

Given that, anything we discuss on medicines, treatments, or doctors is based on discussions we have had with others. We're only qualified to discuss how people might feel about the medical process. To get the facts, our first advice is to buy some books on infertility that address the objective realities of infertility and what treatments are available.

It's Time to Seek Help

You have been trying to get pregnant and still haven't had a baby, or are having trouble having another child. Time has passed, and having children the normal, accepted, way isn't working. If you haven't done so already (and you are a woman), at minimum go to a gynecologist to see if anything is obviously not working properly. Men should see a urologist (more on this later).

Seeing a gynecologist is not a big step. You do this for exactly the same reason that you would see any doctor. If your throat seems tight and sore, you go to the doctor to make sure you don't have an infection. Similarly, you should have a routine gynecological check-up to see if you have an infertility issue that can be resolved quickly. A gynecologist is a professional who can often help you get pregnant and have a baby through standard, non-invasive treatments.

If you don't already have a gynecologist, we advise you contact your local RESOLVE chapter, if you have one. RESOLVE doesn't recommend doctors, but they do keep a list of qualified physicians.

Gynecologists are usually obstetricians as well. It is not easy going into a waiting room with pregnant women when you are having trouble with conception. Your local RESOLVE chapter can inform you of gynecologists in your area who also see infertility patients and who are not obstetricians.

RESOLVE members are very sensitive to women experiencing the pain of infertility, because they either are or have been infertile themselves.

As medical technology continues to advance, more and more infertility treatment is successfully handled by practicing gynecologists/obstetricians (ob/gyn). So you may be pleasantly surprised to learn that your ob/gyn, whom you are already comfortable with, may be able to administer treatments that will help you to have a baby. Be sure to ask what your ob/gyn can do for you.

At minimum, you will probably do some basic tests, like temperature charting or a hormonal workup. You may even begin doing temperature charting on your own. It is simple, and a good indication of whether or not a woman is ovulating. It is a lot of fun taking your temperature every morning before you get up out of bed (I swear!).

You want to start out simple. Hopefully, working with a gynecologist will allow you to become pregnant. It works most of the time. Thankfully, the odds are with you in the conception business.

We fervently hope that this is as far as you need to read in this book and that your infertility journey will end quickly, with a healthy baby as a result.

I Need to Go Further — (Gynecologists, Urologists, and Endocrinologists, oh my!)

You may find that your gynecologist makes one of two recommendations: either to continue with more advanced treatments with the gynecologist or to see an infertility specialist to try to figure out why you are not getting pregnant.

Gynecologists are the physicians who normally identify an infertility problem. If you are comfortable with your gynecologist, his or her recommendation to go further should be a good indication that you need to. However, we recommend you consider carefully and solemnly the decision to go further. Ask a lot of questions. At this point, you are about to move beyond less invasive techniques and into treatment areas that will have more impact on your body, your emotions, and your daily schedule.

Suddenly, it really takes more than two to have a baby. The third person involved may still be your gynecologist, or it may be a recommended infertility specialist (reproductive endocrinologist). Either way, you need to make a prudent decision about bringing someone into one of the most intimate parts of your life — the effort to have a baby.

There is no magic and there are very few rules. One specialist might be good for you but wrong for another patient. You obviously need to get someone qualified to do infertility treatment. You also need to make sure you and your spouse are comfortable with the person. You need to be able to talk with your doctor. You need to be able to ask questions and to get answers you can understand. You need someone who doesn't mind spending a little extra time to make sure you do understand. Part of the whole treatment process will be based on things you must do. You will be more comfortable following your doctor's advice if you understand and are comfortable with that advice.

Time Out: Has the Man Been Checked?

Before you go very far into more invasive options, the man needs to be checked for abnormalities in sperm quantity and quality by a urologist who specializes in infertility. In general, the tests for a man are a lot easier and usually less costly than for a woman.

At a minimum, you need to determine if the two of you are "compatible" in your bid to have a baby. You may find that the man has a medical condition that needs to be treated, or that he has an infertility issue that needs to be dealt with. There may be some resistance here, but you have to get past the concept that infertility "is only a woman's issue." It takes two to make a baby, and now that you are about to bring in a third, you need to ensure that the first two are as ready as possible.

As a man, sometimes it's easy to be **too busy** to get yourself checked out. This infertility business is for the wife to work on, right? "If we're having trouble getting pregnant, she needs to take care of it." Or so it seems. In reality, men need to cooperate at this point. We don't think we can say it enough. Get tested yourself! Don't assume all this is only your wife's responsibility. It could be yours. Just think, if she goes through all this medical work and diagnosis and cost, and the reason that you are not getting pregnant is that you are the one who needs treatment, you have just wasted a lot of time and money.

Why start an expensive regimen of treatment on the female side only to find out that a simple procedure on the male side might have resolved the issue?

Decision Time: What to Do, How Far to Go?

Once you have performed the basics and are told you need to do more, do your utmost to make this next step a mutual decision with your spouse. The two of you are in this together, regardless of what the outcome of testing reveals. And remember those marriage vows, for better or worse? This may be a time where only one spouse has a problem with fertility and you as the partner must be supportive, comforting and understanding.

Medical treatment is going to affect you both, even if only one of you is actually taking medication, or getting operated upon. Don't rush into the decision to do advanced treatments. Take a long weekend to talk it over. Set yourself up in a calm, relaxing setting where you won't be interrupted, and where the potential for anxiety is lessened.

You will need as much information as possible when you sit down for this talk with your spouse. Does your insurance cover treatment? Do you have recommendations on what specialists to approach? Do you have suspicions as to why there is a problem, or have evidence of what the problem is? All of these things need to be discussed thoroughly.

You are about to venture into a new direction in your life. You are about to invite someone else into one of the most private parts of your life, the conception of a child.

We won't say "Just relax" at this point, because we ourselves have heard that too often in our quest for a child. But it is important to reach this decision as calmly as possible. This is a decision that is much bigger than buying a house or finding a new job.

There is no doubt that this decision is stressful and you will feel like you do not have all of the information necessary to make an informed decision at this point. However, not staying calm may not add to your pregnancy problems, but it can prevent you from having a decent life. Remember that twenty years down the road, you will have an answer to your infertility issues. If you are always stressed out during this period, you will get your answer, but you will probably get the same answer if you manage to approach the problem as rationally as you possibly can. (And, yes, we know that this is not easy advice to take.)

In approaching the issue in a straightforward, logical way, you may find some revealing discoveries in your search for a baby. Maybe you will realize something as simple as the fact that you are not having sex at the right time or often enough. Maybe you cannot afford to pay for an infertility specialist and you will have to find less expensive methods in your efforts to bring children into your family. Maybe you will learn that your partner doesn't have the same desire for children you do and is not as willing to bring a third person into the process of trying to have a child.

You need to answer for yourself where you are going in the future, how you want to get there, and what you want to achieve as you quest for children. Answers to these questions will help you decide if advanced medical intervention is correct for you.

Ok, I'm Ready. How Do I Choose a Specialist?

If and when the time comes for you to see a specialist, don't forget to read books written by physicians on the current treatments. Be sure the books are up-to-date, because the field is constantly changing. It is hard to keep up with it.

We remember the first RESOLVE meeting we went to, after we had taken some time off from our own treatment. The treatments the others were undergoing and the terms they used confused us. Many of the treatments were the same but their names had changed or been abbreviated. Some of the treatments were brand new since we had been treated. And we thought we had done every treatment possible. Wrong! Infertility treatment is a young field and physicians and researchers are learning every day.

Determine the category of your infertility if you can. This will help you choose your doctor based on specialty. For example, if you have had your tubes tied previously or have had a vasectomy you will be in quite a different category than someone with undiagnosed infertility.

We found our first reproductive endocrinologist by asking friends in the medical profession who they thought was good in this field. When the same name came up several times, we decided to seek an appointment with him and receive treatment. Remember, most women experiencing infertility are generally healthy, just unable to conceive and/or carry a child to term without medical help. You can take a little bit of time and choose who you see. It is not a decision that needs to be made in haste.

Choose your doctor carefully. You will need to talk to this doctor about very personal issues, and you will be asked very personal questions that can be embarrassing. Having a doctor you can talk to because he or she is personable and caring, in addition to being an expert helps immensely. The way one of our interviewees described their doctor was: "Our doctor puts you at ease. You just know you will get pregnant, because she helps you to feel you can." This couple did get pregnant and now have a son.

The first time you see a doctor, consider yourself to be interviewing them. Think about it. Your choice of doctor is more important than the one you make when interviewing for a job. Our reproductive endocrinologist was always positive about our being able to conceive. He wasn't guaranteeing us a pregnancy, but he did give us hope.

We have also found that knowing some of the medical science of conception before going to a specialist can help. That is why reading some current infertility books on the medical side of infertility is so important. You enter into the physician/patient relationship with a better understanding of what you expect to happen and are expected to do. You are better able to ask knowledgeable questions and make more informed decisions. In addition, your stress is reduced, because you are not always wondering what is happening to your body. If you educate yourself and the doctor further educates you, you are not guessing about the treatment process in addition to worrying how soon you will get pregnant.

If you think you have made a mistake in the choice of your infertility specialist, choose again. This is not like buying a house you find you do not like but must keep. You need to be sure you are able to work with your specialist and he or she can work with you. We had to make the hard decision to switch from one doctor to another doctor. At first we felt we were being disloyal, but after we switched, we knew it had been the right decision.

Your doctor is not God. Yes, the doctor is going to try to help you to do something that seems Godlike — bringing new life into the world.

Some people have too much faith in their doctors, somehow forgetting that they are human also. Thus, even if the doctor won't explain things to them or doesn't appear to truly understand how to help in their particular situation, people continue to see that doctor, hoping for a miracle.

Every reproductive endocrinologist we have worked with told us that infertility is usually solved by persistence. You will spend a lot of time working with your doctor. If you feel your doctor is not meeting your needs, bring it up. There may be a small communication problem that can easily be fixed. But, if you can't resolve the problem, you should probably seek another physician.

On the flip side, you don't want to go from doctor to doctor just because something didn't work right one particular time. Treatment for infertility sometimes works simply through sheer persistence. Sometimes you need to stay with the same doctor because his or her methods work; it just takes time. No doctor will be able to help every one of his or her patients. There will be successes and failures. That is why a good working relationship with your doctor is so important.

Make your choice carefully. This is your future life and family we are talking about!

— Seeking Help, Choosing a Doctor —

The Bookstore

I decided to take action. We've been trying to have a baby for a year, and nothing has happened. My gynecologist says that everything seems okay, but she thinks that I should see a specialist.

That's fine, but now that I'm in this *infertile* category, I'm not about to go into it unaware. I have a friend, Sally, who tried for five years before she finally had a son via IVF. At the time, I didn't even know what IVF was. Sally told me that what helped her most were the books on how to get pregnant. After reading them, she'd know what the doctor was talking about. Sometimes she felt she knew as much as the doctor. That helped keep her confidence up and also made her feel that she was really making progress toward having her baby.

That sounded right to me. I'm a voracious reader, and knowing what was coming seemed the only sensible way to go. So, I went to the bookstore to look for infertility books and publishers of self-help books. I didn't initially find anything in the self-help section, so I kept searching for the infertility section. I finally found a small label saying **Fertility** under the parenting books.

The parenting section had sixteen shelves, thirty-four inches wide, of books discussing the parenting of young children. Eight more shelves were on pregnancy, birth, and preparing yourself for pregnancy. At the very bottom there was a half shelf, eighteen inches, of books on infertility. As I said, the shelf was positively labeled **Fertility**. The other side of the aisle I was in featured the beginning of children's books. The bright, cheery titles were the ones I wanted to read to my child some day when they were four to six years old.

The books were virtually on the floor, so I decided to join them. I plopped down on the carpet in order to better be able to go through the titles. I was happy to find the books Sally recommended. I was also pleased to find that the publication dates were recent, showing they'd been updated to reflect recent findings. I also pulled out four books on the emotional aspects of infertility. Just as doctors wrote the medical books, these were all written by counseling professionals. To be expected, I guess.

I put the emotional books back. I hoped I'd never get to the point where I'd need those! At this point, all I needed to do was read the medical books, get a good specialist, and I'd have a baby within a year. Sure, I was a little frazzled because I'd already been trying a year, but I wasn't nearly as bad as Sally had been during her frustrating medical work-ups.

I'd picked out three of the medical books to buy when a toddler came into the aisle. He was happily pointing to one of the children's books with a picture of Peter Rabbit on the cover. His mother quickly appeared. I said to myself, "Didn't you just know she was going to be seven months pregnant?"

Sitting on the floor, I smiled at both of them as I tried to hide the titles I was looking at. While the little boy kept trying to get his mother to look at the Peter Rabbit book, she was doing a little dance to keep from stepping on either her son or me.

She was looking at the middle shelf, pulling books like *Your Pregnancy Week by Week*; *Breast Feeding Your Baby*; *What to Expect When You're Expecting*; and *Welcoming Your Second Baby*. She was quite friendly, explaining that she was really looking for books for her pregnant friend, and that the book on the second baby was for her.

She never questioned why I was sitting on the floor; she was probably grateful that I looked at the Peter Rabbit book with her son while she explored the parenting books. At his level, I must have been less threatening, because he kept running and pulling more books for me to look at.

They finally left, and I picked up my guilty load of three medical books. I don't know why I didn't leave earlier. I had already finished when they arrived. I looked mid-shelf at the parenting books. A really cute infant looked back at me. Another book cover featured a cartoon couple with two kids and a title above saying, "If we'd wanted quiet, we wouldn't have had children!"

My business instinct had to applaud the bookstore for placing these titles mid-shelf. The covers were great, enticing you to buy. Also, if you were pregnant, you couldn't get down on the floor like I could. The bookstore was definitely in business to sell books and a good display helps. I have to admit that if I had been in the market to buy a book on pregnancy, child birthing or child rearing, these displayed covers would be tempting.

On the other hand, it bothered me that I had to be in the parenting and children's section while looking for infertility books. Okay, I'll admit it. It was discouraging! I was the department manager for women's clothing at a major retail store, and I'd never put size six next to size twenty-four.

My curiosity was piqued, so I asked to see the store manager. I wanted to know how they decided to categorize these books. A very pleasant woman came out to talk to me. I showed her the section, pointing out the title of parenting and then where the infertility books were. I admitted that the parenting books would be more popular, and should indeed be on the higher shelves, but suggested that having the fertility books on the lowest shelf was somewhat demoralizing. I suggested that maybe they would be better off in the self-help section. After all, that's where I had looked first.

The manager listened carefully and admitted that some stores put them in the health section. She tried to be sympathetic, but explained that she felt the parenting section was correct, pointing out that was where I had looked second. She noted that I had not considered the health section, and fertility books were about trying to be a parent. She thanked me for my candid feedback and said that she did understand where I was coming from.

Even though her justification sounded good, I walked away depressed. As a department manager, I knew she had said the things she should to keep a customer satisfied. I couldn't guess how she really felt.

Somehow, I felt that by putting the books in parenting, the store was assuming that all infertile couples would end up having children. And I would! But I didn't have a child yet, and that made it discouraging. I walked back over to the aisle and looked at the emotional books again. One was written by a counselor who had encountered infertility herself. I added that to the three medical books I had already decided to buy. I crossed my fingers, hoping that reading the medical books and getting a specialist would be enough. But you never know — maybe this extra book would help me, even now.

— Handling Drugs and Surgery —

Treatment: Blessing or Curse?

Have you bought some books on how to get pregnant yet? Books that discuss current terminology and show how technology will help provide that baby you long for? If not, do. There are some good, up-to-date medical books written by infertility doctors.

We are not trying to compete with them about what treatments you should pursue to get pregnant. As we said earlier, we are not medical authorities. However, having experienced medical infertility treatments over the course of numerous years, we can discuss what you will encounter in general terms.

Most follow a logical progression in the medical treatment of infertility. First you must admit that you need to do something about your infertility. You start with your ob/gyn and then, if referred, a specialist. Once you begin medical treatment, it can be both costly and life changing. However, a medical diagnosis of the problems you are experiencing and an understanding of when you are most fertile can sometimes help you achieve results without prolonged medical treatment.

So in the first step of getting a medical diagnosis, your gynecologist, reproductive endocrinologist, or urologist will play detective. Specifically, they need to answer the following question: Is the problem of conception inherent to the man, the woman or to both?

Certain reproductive biological systems must be working in a specific manner when you are trying to conceive. When a pregnancy is not occurring; doctors try to find out what is not working properly or is inefficient enough to make conception difficult. The diagnosis process can be extensive.

Sometimes a problem can be remedied with corrective surgery. For example, a woman may have a problem like endometriosis or adhesions. A woman may need a reversal of a tubal ligation or the man, a vasectomy. The man may have a varicocele.

When there is not an obvious problem or indicated surgery, usually the doctor asks the woman to take her basal temperature every morning to see if ovulation is occurring. Assuming that the woman is ovulating, the next step is to test the sperm of the man. These very simple tests indicate if the basics of conception are working.

The diagnostic profile for men is much simpler and less invasive than for women. A urologist specializing in infertility typically examines men for male infertility. We suggest getting a referral from a gynecologist you trust. There are standard tests to examine sperm quality, morphology and motility. As with most situations, if the urologist recommends surgery, get a second opinion.

The next step in this sometimes complex dance of conception and birth, assuming the man checked out fine, is to do some simple testing on the woman to evaluate what the problems are and then possibly more testing to determine how these problems can be fixed or circumvented.

The good news is that most problems can be treated successfully today.

The most common treatments for infertility are drugs that increase the development and release of eggs each cycle or that increase the man's sperm count.

Women are born with the same number of eggs they will have for their entire life. These eggs are the same age as the woman. Eggs age, with a greater failure rate for older women. Sometimes this is the problem that needs solving. That is, fertility drugs help a woman produce a larger quantity of mature eggs per cycle instead of just one or none. It is easy to understand how a woman producing more mature eggs per cycle would have a greater chance of success than if only one egg is produced.

The possibility of multiple births can be scary, even when you desperately want at least one baby. This is where that good relationship with your doctor is critical. If you feel comfortable questioning your doctor, you will have the answers you need to make the right decisions for you and your spouse.

These drugs, although necessary to increase fertility, also have side effects you will need to be aware of and to deal with. Your doctor and pharmacist can help you learn what the side effects might be.

We also strongly recommend that you seek out others undergoing similar treatments for information and support. You could use the "pep rally." The organization RESOLVE is one avenue; there may be other similar support groups in your area as well. A friend going through the process is another avenue. The Internet is a powerful way to converse with people in similar situations. You also can meet people at the doctor's office when you go in for treatments who might become comrades as well. You don't have to experience this alone unless you choose to do so.

One of the worst days for side effects for the woman is the day you start your period. You empower these drugs with the ability to help you get pregnant, so when they don't work, you feel betrayed. You wonder why you went through all of this effort when nothing happened. You're ready to quit. You don't see that magical moment in your mind of you and your spouse holding your baby and the world being filled with music and rainbows. You see only darkness and feel barren. You question who you are and what you are worth if you can't get pregnant. You feel cursed.

During the next few days or maybe the next week you will decide to try again, but right then you often feel that there is no way you would ever do it again. You cry. You weep. Life is such a disappointment. It is then that you need to pamper yourself with a long bath, a new book, an article of clothing, or a nice relaxing dinner with your spouse. You need to get your mind off of the problem. You need to do something that makes life worthwhile again.

It is important to remember that you are both hurting. Even if your husband is not worried about the cycle not working in a given month, he is worried about how this failure to conceive is affecting you. Take time to discuss your feelings. It can help.

During treatments, make sure you eat right, take your vitamins, get lots of sleep and try to exercise moderately. Although you can get pregnant when you are not healthy, try to be as healthy as possible, both for your chances to get pregnant and for your own sake.

If you are in a situation where the drug therapy is beginning to diminish the quality of your life, we recommend keeping in focus what this is all about — a healthy baby of your own to hold and to nurture. Focusing your thoughts on the end goal is the biggest thing to help you through the side effects. Some days you have to remind yourself often that there is a magnificent end goal if you can finish running the race.

The struggle is to be as persistent with the treatments as possible so you can become pregnant. We are referring here to staying in the treatments for the long run, not to having treatments every month. Sometimes you may need to take time off from the schedules and drugs. You need to stay healthy. You need time to be who you are in life. It is hard to do this when you are always following a pre-set course of "when to do what" so you might conceive.

Medical treatment of infertility is hard, time-consuming, costly and schedule-driven. One loses modesty. One also loses naive beliefs like one can conceive any time one wants, and that one controls their own fertility. For many people, this loss of control is one of the biggest losses and disappointments.

Most infertile couples are eventually able to hold a biological child of their own even if it means struggling for years, going through numerous treatments, and suffering the anguish of infertility.

— Handling Drugs and Surgery —

Interruptions

It was 5:03 A.M. Roy slowly put on his coat and tie while thinking about the events of the last half hour. When had lovemaking turned into a ritual? Teri had jostled him awake at about 4:30am, reminding him that it was time to make love.

She wasn't really waking him up because she wanted to, of course. Nor was he in the mood. But it was that time of the month again – the time when she was to be artificially inseminated in a doctor's office. Roy felt like a lab animal – they needed his sperm, someway, somehow.

Teri was trying to be nice about it, of course. She thought that by making love, it would be easier. Even if he had to "pull back" – right at that most important point, and put his sperm into a plastic cup instead of where it belonged, in his opinion: in her, to make a baby.

Roy appreciated the "making love" gesture by Teri, even if he didn't think much of the pain they were currently going through. He wanted a child as much as Teri. But the constant demands on both of them were wearing quite thin.

Roy stared at the little plastic cup containing his sperm. "I hope you're worth it," he said, to the bottle. Lovemaking had stopped being fun. It had become a chore. And he didn't really like that.

The clock was pronouncing 5:13 A.M. when Roy re-entered the bedroom. He was now formally dressed in his business uniform and was beginning to pull on his overcoat. Although Teri appeared to be asleep again, he jostled her awake and said, "It snowed last night. And it's *cold* outside. What do I do with the sperm sample? Didn't the doctor say not to let it get cold?"

Teri pulled up the covers tightly around her. She said, "The doctor said to put it between your breasts. That'll keep it warm. Thanks for letting me sleep another hour."

Roy muttered to himself, "That would work better for you than me." Nonetheless, he took the sample cup and placed it under his overcoat. He held it in place with his left hand, and braved the icy steps with only one hand to keep his balance. He drove to the doctor's office, diligently arriving by 5:35 A.M. He dropped off the sperm sample, and carefully placed both his and Teri's name on the sample. God forbid that they'd ever mix it up with someone else's.

As usual, Roy decided he might as well go into work. The company watchmen always stared at him when he arrived this early, but he never bothered to explain his actions to them.

At 7:00 A.M., Teri arrived at the doctor's. She always wanted to get this over with as soon as possible. As head of her accounting department, she didn't have trouble being late to work, but it usually meant that she worked late those nights. Finally, about 8:30 A.M., the nurse beckoned her in.

Teri removed her dress and panties and climbed up on the chair she referred to herself as the crotch spreader. As a teenager, she would have been appalled at the fact that she exposed herself like this, but now it seemed a regular event.

The doctor came in and made some small talk as he prepared the sample. Both the doctor and Teri tried to ignore what was actually going on, but this time Teri seemed acutely aware of the event. How could things have gotten to the point where she would let a stranger spread her vagina, stick a cold instrument up her, and spray sperm into her body? It was unnatural. It was disgusting. It was ... something that happened over and over.

Afterwards, Teri got into her car, drove to work, and acted as if nothing had happened. Nothing at all; other than being late to work once again.

Trying to Get Pregnant

◇ ◇ ◇

"You'd think that with all this money we've spent, something would happen!" cried Teri. She was staring at her computer screen, trying to argue with Quicken that she and Roy must have more money than the program was saying. She flipped over to Excel to look at her temperature charts, but even the normal comfort of numbers didn't help when all the numbers signaled negative.

"She's on her period, she's on her period," thought Roy to himself, over and over as a mantra. He knew that almost anything would set her off at this point. It had been that way ever since she started on the Pergonal. The fact that nothing was happening even with the Pergonal didn't help at all. "Honey, I know it's been three times, but next time it'll work. The doctor seems optimistic. Look, why don't we go ahead and tap into the European trip money; you're worth it."

"Where do you think I've been taking the money from to pay for the first three times?" Teri screamed. She typed furiously on the keyboard, and brought up the European account balance. The program happily complied, displaying $72.44 as the total funds available to go to Europe.

"What?" asked Roy in disbelief. "We've been saving for this trip for over three years."

"And that's how quickly it goes, too. And nothing to show for it!" Teri started banging on the keyboard. Quicken protested with beeps and clicks, and tried to be helpful by bringing up the new check screen.

Roy pulled her hands away from the computer and held her. Teri started bawling, and Roy wasn't far behind. All that money gone. And only a crying wife to show for it. Europe looked further away than ever.

"We can't afford another cycle." Teri murmured into Roy's chest. Of course, this cycle would be the one that worked. The same was true of the last cycle, until it had passed.

"We can borrow the money from your mother," suggested Roy carefully, afraid of causing another outburst. Teri and her mother didn't get along very well, and money borrowed from her mother usually came easily, but with emotional strings attached.

But all Teri said was, "Ok. But just this once. It has to work this time."

✧ ✧ ✧

The dining room table was elegantly set. The twelve tea settings were all in place; everything was prepared for the Saturday tea. The guest lecturer was in town, and the two months of planning that Teri had put into this event were finally coming to fruition. She hadn't been able to do this type of event in quite a while, but Pergonal shots were not going to prevent this get-together from being perfect.

"Brrrinng!" the phone asked for attention. Teri picked it up quickly, hoping that the person calling wasn't canceling.

"Hi, honey," greeted Teri's mother. "Is everything ok?"

"Yes, mother. I'm about to have a nice tea and talk with some friends."

"That's nice. I just called to see how you were, but I wanted to ask a question. Roy said that the money I sent to you last week was to help you get pregnant, and of course I want that as much as you do. But he mentioned something about a Pergonal test or exam or something and I was reading an article in the paper. You aren't taking this Pergonal thingy, are you?"

"Well, yes, mother, taking Pergonal shots is what helps my eggs to develop," offered Teri cautiously.

"Oh, my. Oh, my. That Pergonal causes you to have a litter of children! Didn't you know that's how those septuplets were born? You don't want that! Your baby brothers Jimmy and Joe were twins, and Lord knows, they're still a handful. I didn't send you my money so you could ruin your lives by having a litter like dogs and cats do!"

Teri's mother heard Teri begin to choke up. "There, there, honey, I didn't mean to make you feel bad. It's just that I wanted to make sure you knew what you were getting into. It's ok if you want to have children. You just don't want too many at once! I'm really concerned about you and Roy. I've been reading lots of stuff on this subject. If you *do* get pregnant, and you have too many kids, you can always do this thing called pregnancy reduction. If you have five or six in your tummy, you can pick the best one or two and get rid of the extras. Oh, honey, don't cry. I'm just trying to help!"

"I know, mother, I know," Teri sobbed. "Don't worry; I won't have more than two. I'll be lucky if I can have one."

"Well, honey, you have a nice tea. You know I only want the best for you and Roy." The phone clicked and Teri was alone again with her thoughts. She allowed herself to slide down the kitchen cabinet until she sat on the floor. The phone started chanting "bedeep, bedeep, bedeep" as an entreaty to be hung up. Teri let the handset fall to the floor.

"Ding dong!" merrily sounded the doorbell. "Damn!" was the only word that came into Teri's head. "What now? Oh, no, the tea party."

Teri jumped up from the floor and rushed to the door. She opened it to the smiling face of her best friend, Diana. "Oh, thank God!" said Teri. Teri rushed Diana into the house and immediately began crying.

"It's these stupid drugs!" stammered Teri. "I'm not this emotional, I'm not!"

Diana managed to get the story of the phone call out of Teri. Teri continued to cry and say, "Why does the world make this happen?" Diana hugged Teri and patted her shoulder. She realized that Teri was in no condition to have a tea party.

"You go upstairs and lie down. I'll run the party for you. After all, Dr. Plodkin will be doing most of the talking. She'll keep everyone entertained. You don't even have to be here. If you want to come down, fine, but don't feel you have to. I'll run it, ok?" Diana spoke softly, hoping to soothe Teri. She took a tissue to wipe the makeup and tears that were running down Teri's face.

Teri just said, "Ok," and allowed herself to be led upstairs to the bedroom where Diana proceeded to remove Teri's shoes and put her in bed. Finally, Diana turned on the ceiling fan to block out the downstairs noise and quietly closed the bedroom door. Then she went back downstairs, hung up the phone, and awaited Teri's guests.

✧ ✧ ✧

"Sweetheart! I'm home! And guess what? Mr. Stoneman and his wife have invited us to go to 'Les Miserables' with them tonight at the Lion Theatre. This is my chance to make an impression, and boy am I proud to have you there with me!" Roy almost bubbled as he walked into the house.

"But, but, tonight is an HCG shot. It has to be precisely at 8:30 P.M., you know that! We can't go, where would I get you to give me the shot?" Teri was in the middle of trying to start dinner, as she herself had just gotten home from work.

"We can find some place to do it at the Lion. I've given you the Pergonal and HCG shots now for almost four cycles; we can do it somewhere other than our bathroom. And this is a good chance to get to know the Stonemans better!" entreated Roy.

A hurried dinner, a quick dressing for the theatre. "Why tonight?" thought Teri. "Why not some advance warning?" She bundled together the syringe, the needle, and the HCG. Almost without thinking, she packed two of each. She put on her lipstick and a nice set of pearls. Roy kept looking at his watch muttering, "We'll be late, we'll be late."

Teri had to admit that they had fantastic seats. But all she could think about was her 8:30 performance. The play started at 8:00 P.M., so she kept trying to think when would be appropriate to take a quick leave of absence. At the end of a song? A lull?

Roy seemed to have forgotten all about the HCG shot in trying to make an impression. The play started, and Teri almost had to jab Roy with an elbow at 8:20 P.M. "Let's go!" she hissed.

"Ok, ok," said Roy. He turned to the Stonemans and whispered, "We'll be right back. Teri has to get her medicine."

Teri was immediately embarrassed, but not enough to keep her from grabbing Roy's hand and sneaking up the aisle. In the background, the musical words of Fantine ground into her memory:

Trying to Get Pregnant

> *"I dreamed a dream in time gone by,*
> *when hope was high and life worth living.*
> *I dreamed that love would never die;*
> *I dreamed that God would be forgiving.*
> *Then I was young and unafraid,*
> *and dreams were made and used and wasted.*
> *There was no ransom to be paid,*
> *No song unsung, no wine untasted.*
> *But the tigers come at night,*
> *with their voices soft as thunder.*
> *As they tear your hopes apart,*
> *as they turn your dream to shame."*

The entrance doors to the auditorium mercifully quieted Fantine's voice. Teri said, "Ok, Mr. Smarty-Pants, where do we do this?"

"The bathrooms should be empty now that the play has started," said Roy confidently. But they soon found that wasn't the case; they were both surprised that there was considerable activity in the lobby and the bathrooms even given that the play was in progress. "Why aren't they watching the play?" pondered Roy.

"It's 8:40 P.M.! I know there is *some* flexibility around these shots, but the doctor made it clear that we need to do it for everything to work right." Teri was getting frantic. Roy was concerned she'd break down again right in the theatre. Then what would he say to the Stonemans?

"Ok!" said Roy. He and Teri were off the lobby near the bathrooms. Roy started trying different doors. "Here's a room!" he said, as one door opened to a janitorial closet. They both rushed into the dingy room lit by a single light bulb. Roy closed the door and surveyed the scene.

Deep sink. Mops. Something that looked like an air-conditioning unit. Tiled floor. "Ugh," thought Teri, but she immediately lifted up her dress and dropped her panties. "Just get it over with!" she said.

Roy fumbled with the medical kit Teri had packed. He pulled out the syringe and needle and tried to put the shot together. In doing so, he fumbled, and the HCG vial dropped to the floor and smashed. "Damn!"

"Thank God, I brought two," muttered Teri. "Use the other one. I don't care. Just do it. Don't you *dare* break this one."

Roy successfully assembled the HCG shot and flicked the syringe with his finger to make sure there were no air bubbles, then turned and saw Teri leaning over the deep sink with her bare behind pointed at him. At one point in his life, Roy had fantasies of making love in very strange places. Now, in a janitor's closet at the Lion Theatre during a performance of 'Les Miserables', all he could think of was, "poke her butt like it was an orange; poke her butt like it was an orange," as he had been taught by the nurses.

The shot itself took only a moment. Teri hiked up her panties, dropped her dress, and said, "Let's get the hell out of here." Roy opened the door, looked both ways, and the two quickly exited.

They re-entered the theatre. Once again, Fantine was singing, but this time they were oblivious to it as they tried to quickly reach their seats. Roy quietly said, "Sorry, it's a medical thing." Teri glared at Roy. For the rest of the play, the actors on the stage were not the only ones who were 'Les Miserables'.

❖ ❖ ❖

The alarm clock chirped happily. "4:30 A.M." stared Roy in the face. "Why did I ever think a bird chirp would be better than an alarm?" he thought, slamming his hand over the clock to silence it.

"That's right," he remembered. Today is sperm sample day. He yawned, wishing for more sleep. Their lives had become one interruption after another, revolving around drugs, doctor visits, and their efforts to become pregnant.

Roy looked over at Teri. Somehow, she had managed to sleep through the alarm. He appreciated her desire to help in getting the sperm sample. On the other hand, he hated waking her up. "Maybe I'll just do it myself," he thought.

This time, it would work. It had to. They couldn't afford another one. They couldn't keep this up. This had to end. "But," Roy thought, "didn't we say this last time, too?"

— Examining Alternative Pregnancies —

Breaking the Rules

What if you can't get pregnant the *normal* way? What if you can't get pregnant through surgery or drugs?

Maybe you've tried. You've gone through the gamut and still no success. Words like "unable to carry to term," "eggs are too old," and sterile haunt you; but they all mean the same thing: *you can't have kids*. Something is stopping the sperm from meeting the egg and doing the fertility dance.

You have two paths on which you can continue your journey. You can accept your situation, or you can start breaking the traditional societal rules in order to succeed in having a child.

"Traditional societal rules" simply means that society believes there is a mother and a father, children result from their union, and they are raised to adulthood. It's always been that way. The exceptions, like divorce, orphans, adopted children, or extended families have long been factored into society's rules system.

Today's medical technology has allowed alternatives to the traditional means of creating a family, but society isn't usually comfortable with the concept. Because of these medical advances, the unspoken rules have become cloudy.

For example:

- What if a woman can't give birth to children, but has her eggs and husband's sperm implanted into another woman? Is she still the mother?

- What if a man is infertile and his wife uses a donor's sperm to have a child? Is he still the father?

- What if a woman decides to surrogate, using her eggs but another man's sperm, so as to give a baby to an infertile couple? What rights does the surrogate have?

- What if a couple adopts, but DNA results prove a formerly unknown man is the father of the child, and this biological father suddenly initiates a claim for the baby?

- What if a child who has been raised by one family is suddenly shown by medical science to belong to another family? Some switch must have occurred long ago!

Medical science has come a long way to help promote new life. But there is controversy about trying to **beat the system** when it comes to having and raising children because the rules don't fit any more.

The fact that these rules don't adequately address surrogacy, DNA testing, or sperm/egg donors have caused the rules to be reconsidered. Over the last twenty years, the concepts of "mother's rights," "father's rights," "children's rights," "surrogate rights," "adoptive rights," and even "interested parties rights" have all re-entered the debate again, and no clear answers have yet emerged.

We are in a painful transition period where the rules are changing. We see the transition in the courts, where the rules are being redefined, with the new rules sometimes going in one direction, sometimes the opposite. An example is in some adoption cases where the rights of the birth mother are upheld and other adoption cases where the rights of adoptive parents are upheld.

We see the transition in entertainment, with TV programs and movies showing surrogate children, reversed adoption, and babies switched at birth as part of our viewing schedule. Songs by groups like *Heart* deal with having a baby by another man because her own husband can't have one. *All I Wanna Do is Make Love to You* is a strangely interesting song combining infidelity with sperm donorship.

Newspaper articles about children switched at birth. Large groups of people reacting both positively and negatively to a couple having septuplets. Adoptions being turned around. Surrogate mothers changing their minds and wanting *their* children. Grandparents deciding to assert their rights when mothers don't want their children.

Amidst all of this change, we ask, "What is the answer? The *correct* answer?"

As infertile couples, we are stuck in the middle of this controversy, because, in part, we *are* the controversy. In order to have our own children, we are sometimes using medical science to challenge the societal rules about having children. We have every right to do so, but if we choose that path we must face the consequences of challenging societal norms.

These comments are not meant to discourage you from taking this road. In getting to this point, you may already have traveled the road of realization, the road of anguish, the road of surgery or drugs, and other alternative roads. This is simply another road; a road where you must once again decide whether the pain involved will be worth achieving your important goal of having a child.

If you decide to travel this road, we encourage you to pursue it with your desire, your heart, and your will. The rules and logic defining this road are still being written.

Notes

— Examining Alternative Pregnancies —

Beating the System

It all seemed so strange and unusual when I look back. I'm still in disbelief. I can't believe it's happening to us. Surely there is some explanation other than infertility for why I am not pregnant.

I remember being at work and leaving early to see my doctor. I like the gynecologist I had found when we moved. He seemed like somebody I could talk to and get real answers to my questions. Not that I had many questions. After all, I'm pretty normal as these things go, and there is nothing unusual with my mother or her mother.

When Brent and I first started to think about having children, we were excited, but scared. Could we really be parents? Of course, we could! After I went off the birth control pill, we waited, like the doctor said, before trying to get pregnant. For the next six months nothing happened. All of my friends were telling me they got pregnant right away. I guess that's when I started to worry.

That day in the doctor's office began our nightmare. The doctor said that from all initial evidence, there should be no problem in me conceiving. There were lots more tests that could be done to see if there was something abnormal, but since everything seemed normal, the doctor recommended testing Brent first to see if he was ok before putting me through a lot of tests that could become expensive and time consuming.

I sat numbly for a few seconds trying to think of what to say next. Then I began asking questions about what tests they wanted to do on Brent. I suppose part of me was listening, but a part of me was screaming, wondering what would happen if Brent were not normal. What if?

That night I showed Brent the literature from the doctor. Brent was willing to be tested. In looking back I don't think he really thought there was much to worry about. Brent's sperm would be tested and everything would be fine and we would get pregnant next month.

In reality, however, we didn't get pregnant the next month, and his sperm test was bad. There was plenty of fluid, but it did not hold much sperm. We began to get a real education about things we never cared much about and still don't. After all, to have a baby you make love and it happens and you don't really think about all of the science that makes it work.

The specialist we were sent to explained that Brent's sperm count was so low that he could not get me pregnant. We had a few decisions to make. We could use donor sperm. That means we could use some other man's sperm to impregnate me artificially. Or we could remain childfree. There was also another alternative, involving putting Brent on Clomid, but more testing on Brent would be necessary to see if that would be helpful.

In disbelief, we asked if that was all. I wanted Brent's child, not some other man's. I didn't think I could use donor sperm and I didn't think Brent would want me to either. The specialist advised us to go home and think about it. Brent's sperm would be tested in another month to see if his count was better. If it was, maybe there would be another option for us. In the meantime, we needed to avoid hot tubs, hot baths and fevers. All of these kill sperm.

After talking with this doctor, we began having trouble discussing things. I was worried about how Brent felt and he was worried about how I felt. We tried to do what we felt would make the other person happy instead of taking time to sort out our own thoughts or feelings or desires. As a result, soon we began to argue and be impatient with one another. When I look back I realize how horrible it became.

I started to read some of the medical books telling couples how to try to get pregnant. It was in one of these books that I found advice telling couples to evaluate how they felt about being infertile. Until an individual sorts out what he or she feels and wants, the person cannot help a spouse understand what he or she wants.

Trying to Get Pregnant

Brent and I decided to take the advice in the book and started to figure out what each of us wanted. Then we tried to talk about what was important to us. When Brent told me he would not object to a sperm donor, I was shocked. In my mind I was so sure that he would not accept it. This shows how wrong I had been! It also shows how much better it was to listen to what Brent wanted rather than assume what he wanted. I suddenly felt that maybe we would be able to have the children we had both dreamed of. I still wanted Brent's child, but if that could not be, we could at least be parents. There was hope again!

The process wasn't as complicated as we had expected. We had to decide what attributes we wanted in the male donor. We were given profiles of the sperm donor which included such items as hair color, eye color, body type, and education.

Once we choose our donor, artificial insemination was used to get me pregnant. My pregnancy went well; the only problems were those days when I still wondered how Brent felt about this being my baby, but not his. He said over and over that it was our baby. Finally, I think I believed him.

Now, looking at our three-year-old, whom we named William, I wonder where the concern ever was. He looks just like Brent in his baby pictures. He is even getting pretty good at throwing the ball back to Brent when they play toss. Brent's parents tell us all the time how athletically inclined Brent was as a child. They sometimes forget that we had donor sperm, because they compare so many of William's features and abilities to Brent's. He is our baby, not just mine.

It's been wonderful. As I look down at my extended belly, I am so very glad I am a mother, even if it must be achieved through the help of a donor. Soon I'll be the mother of two. And, yes, Brent will be the father of two.

Notes

— Considering Prayer —

Prayer: Can it Help?

So far, we have mainly discussed dealing with the physical issues associated with infertility and trying to get pregnant; doctors, medicines, surgery, eggs, sperm, etc.

But what about the mental and spiritual issues? We get so wrapped up in the physical aspects of getting pregnant that we sometimes neglect the mental and spiritual aspects that may help us get pregnant.

We are not about to say "Just relax, you'll get pregnant." We've heard that so many times that we want to scream! Besides *just* relaxing is not going to get you pregnant. On the other hand, being in a good mental state prepared for the issues of each day and for eventual pregnancy is beneficial to your life and overall well-being. The well-meant *lower your stress, just relax, take it easy* mantras do have some basis. Not in that they will help you get pregnant, but, if achievable, they can improve the quality of your life while trying to get pregnant. (It doesn't make it any easier to hear these things said over and over, of course.)

We'll be the first to jump up and down in the audience and say "Ok, fine. But how do you accomplish this?" The work and worry and effort required to achieve pregnancy can be all-consuming.

Our answer? Prayer. Or, if you are not comfortable with the word prayer because of its religious overtones, use the word meditation, or relaxation.

Prayer, meditation, and relaxation help you focus your energies in one direction. When you are more directed in your thinking; you can take better actions to meet your goal. This is necessary when you go through infertility treatment, as your time becomes very scheduled. If timetables are not adhered to, you can't do any treatment for that particular cycle. Focusing your thoughts and energies through prayer can motivate you to appropriate action.

Prayer can also put you into a positive frame of mind. If you are anxious and fearful that you won't get pregnant, you may not make totally rational decisions. Your quality of life will also be lessened. You have a choice of pursuing treatment as calmly as possible, or you can just become a big bundle of nerves.

Prayer helps you make decisions. In accepting that you aren't pregnant yet, you can decide to seek help from medical science. Or make the opposite decision; that you don't want to pursue surgery or treatment. It can also help you decide how long to continue with what you are currently doing.

In prayer, you are communicating with yourself, in addition to seeking the intervention, guidance, or sympathetic ear of God. If you believe that prayer will invite God to action, you have another aid in your quest to end your infertility. Even so, prayer is an invitation for you to take action yourself as well as to help achieve the goals of your prayer.

If you do not believe that praying will help, it won't. Prayer is based on attitude. We described prayer in different terms, because sometimes as little as a word misinterpreted can prevent you from being in a good frame of mind. If you believe that you will receive benefit from prayer, or meditation, or relaxation, and you look for that benefit, you will often find it.

We believe in the benefits of prayer. It is one of the few things we recommend without reservation as part of your infertility treatments.

— Considering Prayer —

The Patience of John

John sighed as he walked into the house. It had been a long day, and unfortunately it was going to become even longer. As he prayed, he kept asking God, "Why us? Why did Marie have to have endometriosis, and why is my sperm count low, in fact, non existent? Lord, *why us*?"

John and Marie had been married three years to the day the previous Sunday. It had been a good three years, except for the fact that they could not get pregnant. Larry hinted at the anniversary party about it being time to bring some little pastors into the house for training. Everyone laughed. They were a good group. But neither John nor Marie had been able to tell anyone that they had been trying for the last three years and nothing was happening. As their pastor, how could they respect someone who could not have children? How would they ever understand? John's biggest fear was that they would think him less of a man because he could not father children.

Early each morning, during John's quiet time, his first plea to God was to help Marie conceive. Then, feeling guilty about being so selfish, he would ask for wisdom on how to lead the congregation closer to God, to do God's will, for guidance in accepting other people's faults, and how to work with everyone to bring cohesion within the church.

Now, as he took off his shoes, he wondered how he was going to get through the evening. The deacons were coming over later to discuss the celebration for Mother's and Father's Day and the dedication of the new children's wing. It was a big step for their small church. Financially, they had cut building costs, but they needed their community outreach programs to work so the programs would grow. What was the use of a new wing if there were no children to grace it?

But how could he lead a meeting with a happy face and eagerness that should inspire everyone when he had just found out that he was sterile? He found himself amused at the strangeness of the word. He remembered how he learned in biology class what the term really meant and the sterility jokes he used to share with the other boys in his class.

Marie entered the room. She was still his beautiful bride. God had given him someone he could really love. She noticed his down look and in her attempt to comfort and understand, Marie realized the lack of children was hurting him as much as her. She had a woman's meeting at church that kept her from going to the doctor with him and she had just assumed everything would be fine. After all she was probably the problem because of the endometriosis.

Through a face full of tears John told Marie he had a low sperm count. He was sterile. The doctor did not give much hope. He seemed ready to begin using donor sperm instead of trying to find and correct the problem. They could not afford the cost to determine the problem, and using donor sperm was going to be costly as well. It might not work, given Marie's endometriosis. And neither felt comfortable about using donor sperm. It was not right for them.

Sensing John's anguish, Marie asked if she could call off the meeting. There needed to be some time for John to grieve. Serving God did not mean giving until there was nothing left. But John explained this was the only night they had been able to find for the meeting. They had tried several nights and every other night had conflicts. With Mother's Day only three weeks away, they had to get the initial planning started tonight so that the opening of the new children's wing would go well.

"What if you told them?" asked Marie.

"Told them what?" asked John.

"Explain to the deacons about how we have been unable to have children. Surely they will understand. People are supposed to be able to go to Deacons when they need help. Why can't the pastor go to them as well?"

"And tell them I am sterile? Not on your life. They would lose all respect for me and then where would we be? Without a job and on the street! And if the next church asked why I was discharged, I couldn't exactly tell them that I was unable to father children so I was let go, could I?"

When Marie simply asked what answer he had found from prayer, John just sat there. As he thought on the question, John felt that God for some reason seemed to not even hear his plea on this issue. Other prayer requests were granted. Many people had expressed relief and had received answers when Pastor John prayed with or for them. The whole congregation considered him a true Man of Prayer.

So why was God so silent on the most important request in his life? How could he trust God when God ignored him? Weren't children a reward from the Lord as quoted by David in Psalm 127? Why was God withholding his favor? He and Marie would be good parents. Not like some he counseled who were abusive to their children. Sometimes he almost lost all compassion when he saw what some parents did to their little precious gifts from God.

Marie waited for John to speak and when he did not, she gently told him to use her as the problem. It would not be a lie. There was no reason for the deacons to know there were two problems. And if they could accept Marie as having female problems, maybe some day they could accept that John was sterile. They might even have a recommendation for another doctor so they could get a second opinion. It was worth the chance of telling them. Besides, they were going to know something was wrong.

Marie persuaded John to have a bite to eat and they sat before the meal praying to God with tears in their eyes. Together, they asked God to grace their life with a child. And to take away the pain they had when they saw other people with children, when they did not have any.

At 7:30, the deacons began arriving. Marie had gone into the sewing room so she would not have to face them, especially since they would soon know their secret. John had had enough time to compose himself and put on a happy face before the meeting.

After they had all gathered, John opened the meeting in prayer. Then he told them he had something to discuss with them before they discussed the business of the new wing. He started by saying that he and Marie really wanted to have children, but Marie had recently found out that she was not capable of having a baby. He proceeded to say that he was searching his soul for the best way to give sermons for Mother's Day and Father's Day to launch the new children's wing, but in light of this news, he hoped the deacons would allow a substitute pastor to preach the sermons on those days. He and Marie could go home to honor their parents for the day as the excuse for why he would not be there. He ended by saying that he did not want the news about Marie to get out, as he was unsure if they were ready yet to handle the condolences.

Silence pervaded the room as the news sunk in. All ten deacons had a somber expression. John could tell that most of them did not know what to think. He could also see the pain on some of the faces as they considered what they would now say.

Finally, Larry spoke up. As chairman of the deacons, he tended to guide the group well, and he felt he should show the support that his pastor and pastor's wife needed. He expressed his sorrow at this news, and agreed that it would be appropriate for Marie to visit her parents, especially in light of her Mom's recent illness. However, he believed that the pastor should be the guiding spiritual force behind the opening of the new wing on Mother's Day. After all, even though they both hurt, it was not the pastor's problem that caused them to be unable to have children. So, if Marie went to visit her parents, there shouldn't be a problem. Anyway, some of the best sermons came from pain and anguish. Maybe the Lord could use this tragedy to honor His work at this church. It would be hard, but giving the sermon would help the grieving process that they needed to go through.

Chris chimed in next with empty words of condolence. He expressed the fact that it had taken courage to tell them of this difficulty in having children. But he felt that as strong as pastor was in the Lord, he would bless the church with a most powerful sermon. He agreed that some of the best sermons came from pain and loss and anguish. Maybe God intended for the church to be their children and that is why he blessed them with the funds to build the new children's wing.

The faces of the deacons showed they agreed with this train of thought. After all, they were trying to comfort the pastor. It seemed right that maybe God had planned this after all.

Bill spoke next. "I agree with Larry, pastor. You always have sermons that are inspired by God. Larry's right that Marie should visit her parents, but I can see you giving a really soul-wrenching sermon like you usually do. It's not like we are asking Marie to give the sermon. That would be very inconsiderate of us."

John numbly agreed that they were right. He would spend time in prayer asking God to direct his thoughts so the sermon would honor the work God had already done by allowing them to build the new wing. Then he silently prayed for strength to get through the rest of the meeting without crying.

After the deacons left full of plans and good intentions, John told Marie about their decision and how he would have to give the Mother's Day sermon. It was his responsibility before God. He expressed his agreement that she should visit her parents that weekend. But, Marie declined, knowing that John needed her strength. They were in this together. They would conquer the pain with God's help and He would see them through.

The sermon might not have been God-inspired on that Mother's Day when they dedicated the new children's wing, but John did perform well. Within months, the new wing supported the needs of many children. This work and outreach brought many new families into the church.

After much prayer, John and Marie began to accept the role of surrogate parents to the less fortunate children who were encouraged to come. They began to believe that God had called them to guide and counsel children who were not lucky enough for whatever reason to have good parental guidance. Nonetheless, while they continued to help build the new children's programs, they also continued to pray for a child of their own.

When it happened, it came as a surprise to both John and Marie. Julie, one of the new girls to the church, came to them one Sunday evening after church services telling them she was pregnant. Would they adopt her child? She had seen the love Marie had for children as she led the little ones through the play yard. She wanted that love for her child. She knew that at sixteen, she was not going to be able to provide a home or give that love to her child. Would they?

With tears in their eyes, John led the three of them in prayer. Upon his amen, all of them felt that their prayers had indeed been answered. Julie's child would have parents; John and Marie would have the child they wanted to raise.

Part 3
Acknowledging Your Emotions

Riding the Roller Coaster

    Going Up to Hope   121
    Going Down to Despair   123

Never Expect to be in Control

    Those Everyday "Gotcha" Times   127
    Cat's in the Cradle   131

Oh, Those Holidays

    Can Holidays be Holy?   133
    We Won't Be Home for Christmas   137

What We've Lost

    Can You Touch It?   141
    Can You See It?   145

Quote on page 126 is from the nursery rhyme
Rock a bye Baby
attributed to "Mother Goose" in medieval times.

Quote on page 128 is from the song
Butterfly Kisses
written by Bob Carlisle & Randy Thomas
Copyright 1996
Diadem Music Publishing and Polygram International Publishing, Inc.

— Riding the Roller Coaster —

Going Up to Hope

We've been using a "road of infertility" metaphor to explore how it feels to be infertile. It's a nice, calming way to examine the issues associated with infertility, but, in reality, dealing with infertility on a day-to-day basis is more like a roller coaster.

Roller coasters are fun, right? It's exciting climbing that hill, and even though it's scary and you lose your breath as you drop into the depths, you call that exciting as well because the ride will be over soon. But, on the infertility roller coaster, the end of the ride flashes by, but the roller coaster just keeps on going. You can't seem to get off. Up the hill again, and down into the depths again. Those otherwise exciting dives into the depths are now dreaded; you even get queasy as you go toward the top. You feel as if you are in a never-ending episode of *The Twilight Zone*.

Other people get on the roller coaster, take one trip, and get off — with their new baby — saying "isn't this fun?" as they leave. You may tell them how sick you are feeling and how depressed you are getting. Going up and down over and over is not fun! In fact, you don't have time to take all the other rides or see the other fun things in the carnival because all you seem to be doing is riding this roller coaster. You lament your lost time. You lament the fact that you can't seem to have a baby. Each month you try again, but your hopes are dashed when you go down into the depths once more.

During this tumultuous process you don't get much sympathy. Roller coasters are supposed to be fun. You wanted to do this. You are just continuing to have fun riding the roller coaster.

It's not like a death. A death of someone close to us is more like falling off of a cliff. You land; you suffer grievous emotional injury. It takes a long time to recover from that emotional injury. But the death happened to you, you didn't choose to walk off the cliff. Once you hit the bottom after a death, you do have the ability to get up and begin to recover from your emotional injuries. The fall, though extremely severe, is over. There is an ending, one that you cannot change.

As for you on the infertility roller coaster, there is no apparent emotional injury. Your stomach is queasy and your mind is screaming "Why won't this end?" But friends at the fairground wave happily as the coaster zooms by, saying, "Just relax. Have fun! You'll get there!" as you continue to go round and round and round. No one sees the emotional injuries you are suffering from being continually jostled around. They don't see how you are out of control. It is not like you were at the bottom of a cliff, needing to be picked up and tended to.

You go up again. You no longer look forward to it, even though it might yield that long-awaited child. You know what is probably beyond the rise — another long drop into despair and depression.

So why stay on the roller coaster? It does stop. People do get off. Although you say you can't get off, in reality you could at each stop – but it would be without the child you so desperately want. You stay because to get off is even worse than the ride itself. The rest of the fairgrounds of life pale because you have no child to share in the fun. Everyone else got their child on this ride, why were you the one to fail?

You stay on because of hope. You hope that the next ride will be different. Instead of the drop being the pain of loss and emptiness, the drop will be the pain of labor, delivery, and success. You hope that this will be the last ride, and that you won't have to stay on any longer.

Hope is your driving force to continue. Hope makes it all seem worthwhile.

As long as hope remains greater than the effort, work, loss, despair, and depression, you will continue to stay on the roller coaster. Hope keeps you going.

— Riding the Roller Coaster —

Going Down to Despair

Bright rays of light blind me through the shades, interrupting what little sleep I finally managed to get during a night of tossing and turning. I awake alone; my husband has already escaped to his office in the bustling downtown of another life.

No, I find that I am not alone. The dreaded redhead joined me during the night. Inwardly I wail, as I walk to the bathroom to find a box of napkins. Everything had looked so promising this time. But the seepage of red is stark testimony to the inadequacy of my positive thinking.

I take a shower, trying to wash away my disappointment. My tears join the spray; I kneel as sobs rack my body. Once again, the only issue of my body is blood.

I cannot face the world today. I poke at the phone with my fingers; a happy mechanical voice answers, "Thank you for calling the New Hope Library Center. Our hours are ..." I await the beep and then inform the machine that I am sick and will not be able to come in to work.

Then I go to the kitchen. Sitting at the kitchen table, I notice my container of Serophene pills staring at me, mocking my inability to get pregnant even with its help. I grab the container and throw it across the room, where it bounces off the laundry room door and skitters back toward me.

I need some sympathy so I call my husband's office. I'm put on hold because he's busy. He finally answers with "What is it now?" the irritation in his voice clearly indicates that I have once again invaded the sanctity of his career.

"I started my period," I answer, the blunt truth being all I can muster.

"Oh, hey, honey, I'm sorry to hear that. Look, why don't you take the day off as you usually do when you start your period? Fix us that steak marinade for tonight; you know that's my favorite. We can have a quiet dinner, ok? Look, I've got to get back to my meeting. Oh, hey, yeah, since you're taking the day off, could you buy a baby shower gift for Jim Foraker's daughter? It's his first grandchild, so I want to be sure we get her something nice. Take care, honey. Bye."

The phone goes silent. I place the handle gently into its cradle wondering why I bothered to call. He doesn't care if we have a child. He already has two big strapping boys who visit on weekends. At thirty-five, he can proudly point to his two teenagers on the high school football field. Here I am, at twenty-nine, having to pick up after two boys with their father's face whenever they visit. They call me Mary; Mom is who they live with.

I work up enough energy to go to the store. Unlike the library where I work, no one will ask me how I feel here. I pray I won't run into somebody I know. Unable to muster enough reserves to go to more than one place, I choose the super-store. After purchasing flank steak and other ingredients for dinner, I gird up my bloodstained loins as I head for the baby department.

I bite my lip and try to ignore all the reminders of babies around me. I pick out an obviously expensive baby blanket knowing that my husband would prefer to exhibit the expense over the item. I make the purchase quickly so that I may flee the store.

Home again, and it is noon already. I pull out the flank steak, my wooden cutting board, and the tenderizing mallet. As I pound the strips of steak, my eyes drift to the shopping bags. The baby blanket box says "blessed warmth and comfort" on the side with a picture of a sleeping child haunting me.

I pound the steak with more intensity. The steak becomes the object of my wrath as I beat it. And beat it. And beat it! Utterly subdued, the steak exhibits its tenderized dimples to me as it surrenders to my hammering.

The phone rings and I jump within my seat. It's the library. "On your period again?" asks my nosy co-worker. "It must be nice to take a day off every month." I listen to her blather on the speakerphone as I drown the steak in the marinade.

The food in the fridge, I finally have a few moments to benefit from my temporary escape from the world. I walk downstairs and into my husband's play room, his gigantic home theater. Even a 61-inch screen is not enough for him — he and his boys deserve the best — so with a projection console mounted in the ceiling we now have a full wall theater.

I turn on the system hoping to find a good old movie. Instead a giant baby's head smiles at me. I quickly switch the channel only to be greeted by some show host interviewing "women who threw their babies into trash cans."

The theater system screeches in protest as I shut it down improperly. I don't have much energy, but I have to let out my anger and frustration, so I wander into the second of my husband's playrooms, hoping to exercise my troubles away. I mount the walker and place it on a low setting. I slowly walk as I gaze at my husband's past glories, his football trophies from his college days. I stand as one with them, another statue in my husband's collection.

It seems to take no time at all to work up a sweat, yet I suddenly realize that it is already 4:30. Wiping the sweat from my brow, I walk upstairs to take a shower before replacing the evidence of my barrenness.

As I start preparing dinner, I decide to open one of our special bottles of wine and pour myself a glass hoping my husband won't yell at me for doing so. "It had to breathe," I'll insist. I drink a glass too quickly as I continue to prepare the meal.

Then I call my friend Charlene to get that one ingredient I always forget to add to the steak recipe. In the course of our conversation, she reassures me that I'll get pregnant next month, adding that I'm too hyper about all this and I'll probably be sorry once I have kids and get tired of them.

It's now 7:00 P.M. My husband always gets home about now. The table is set. The wine is poured. I've even put on a nice dress. He always likes that. And I need him to like that.

At 7:10 P.M., I'm looking out the window. He's always on time. As I return to the kitchen, I notice the phone answering machine merrily blinking. "When did I miss a call?" I wonder.

"Hi honey. I guess the phone's busy and I got transferred to the machine. I'm sorry to tell you on such short notice, but Foraker wants me to wine and dine some important clients. So cancel that steak dinner. I'll be home late, so don't wait up for me. Bye." The machine then mechanically intones, "Thursday, 5:27 P.M."

Oh why did I have to be in the shower when his phone call came, I lament.

Reluctantly I eat my steak supper — I don't even like steak — and I drink my own glass of wine as well as his. Then I take his plate and give it to the great beast my husband keeps on a chain out back. He gulps down my day's efforts without as much as a thank you.

I finally come back inside and sit on the couch. I cradle my arms together and very silently sing to the invisible child in my arms before falling asleep amid my tears.

> *"Rock-a-bye, baby in the treetop.*
> *When the wind blows the cradle will rock.*
> *When the bough breaks the cradle will fall.*
> *And down will come baby cradle and all."*

— Never Expect to be in Control —

Those Everyday "Gotcha" Times

You're just living your life, not even thinking about infertility, then, when you least of all expect it, you see a commercial about babies, or hear a song crooning about families, or have a stray thought cross your mind. Your throat catches, tears come into your eyes, and you wonder why you are still struggling to have children.

"Gotcha."

It happens more often than you care to admit, whether you are a man or a woman. It's amazing how quickly it can steal away your composure. You turn away if you are in a group, you try to think about something else, or you let it continue to have a hold on you. Your world is turned upside down just on a word, or a tune, or a memory.

What triggers the "gotcha" varies. It depends on the issues that most bother a person about infertility. But the "gotchas" are there, and will get you when you least expect.

When they come out of hiding, they steal away control of your life, even if only in increments, in moments. They wait at the periphery of your mind.

✧ ✧ ✧

Have you ever heard the song *Butterfly Kisses*? It's a beautiful song, but it's very hard for someone like me to hear. I just played it, but I probably shouldn't have. It's hard to type through tears.

> *Butterfly kisses after bedtime prayer.*
> *Stickin' little white flowers all up in her hair.*
> *"Walk beside the pony*
> *daddy, it's my first ride."*
> *"I know the cake looks funny,*
> *daddy, but I sure tried."*
> *Oh, with all that I've done wrong,*
> *I must have done something right*
> *To deserve a hug every morning*
> *And butterfly kisses at night.*

For a man who longs for a daughter, it's tough to hear this song. I want to do all the things Bob Carlisle sings about. I imagine myself with my daughter. The anticipation rises, then I hear the part about "With all that I've done wrong, I must have done something right to deserve …" The tears come. What have I done wrong so that I don't deserve this?

"Gotcha."

Taking a more sober look, I realize that he's not singing about birth. He's not singing about the existence of his daughter. His daughter's existence was a gift, a privilege. He's singing about deserving the hug, deserving the love of his child. He has done something right in helping to shape her attitudes in life.

Despite this realization, a "Gotcha" nevertheless took my control away.

✧ ✧ ✧

Have you ever equipped a nursery? Have you bought a crib, baby items, or a rocker? Imagine having done so, but that three years have passed in your infertility struggle and you now have to move to another city.

You decide to have a moving sale to sell items you don't need. The two large rockers would be nice when you finally have children, but for now they've become a burden as well as a constant reminder.

So you reluctantly put them out with all of the rest of the stuff you can part with. When you invite friends and family to come by first in case

Acknowledging Your Emotions

they want some of these items, sure enough, your parents decide to purchase the rockers — after all, they are in perfect condition; you've never been able to use them.

A few months later, you return to visit your family. You know that your sister-in-law gave birth recently, and another sister-in-law is due in three months. That's part of life in the infertility world; you know that everyone else has babies. But somehow, you didn't expect to walk into your parents' house and see your sister-in-law with her three-month-old child in your rocker trying to get the baby to go to sleep.

"Gotcha."

No, it wasn't intentional. It wasn't meant to hurt you. In your heart, you know that it is good that the rockers are finally being used for the very reason you purchased them. But it isn't you in the rocker with your child.

✧ ✧ ✧

Men aren't supposed to care. But some men get a lump in their throat as they drive by a playground and see children outside playing. They get tears in their eyes when listening to a song talking about daughters and sons. Luckily, they are alone in the car, and no one has to see them show their emotions.

If they read something in the newspaper about how the best word in the world is "Daddy," they may pull the paper up higher in front of them to hide their faces until they regain their composure by reading about some foreign conflict. If they watch a movie like *Finding Nemo*, they'll pretend that none of the Father/Son scenes affected them.

The reason men don't seem to care is that they hide how they feel. That is, those "gotchas" usually can be disguised. And usually, men avoid situations where they might have to show how they feel.

So imagine how a man might feel in seeing a movie about a grown-up Peter Pan. When Peter needs to be able to fly again to save the day, he has to think about his "happy thought" in order to do so. And his happy thought is ... the birth of his first-born son.

"Gotcha."

It's embarrassing for a man to break down crying in the middle of a large movie theater right when the hero begins to save the day.

❖ ❖ ❖

Infertility seems so pervasive. Everywhere you turn there seems to be reminders that you are different. You have not had children.

If you love to sew, it is hard to walk into a fabric store, when all the walls are covered with patterned fabrics for making baby quilts, with bears and bunnies in soft pastels. You can't make them. It would be too painful to stare at Winnie the Pooh for hours as you finish the project.

But one day a friend who is expecting finally takes you up on your gift offer by requesting a baby quilt. You focus on how useful the quilt will be and how much it will be used and enjoyed. You do everything you can to concentrate on what the quilt is for instead of why you don't make one for yourself.

After many hours of work, you present the baby quilt to your friend. She loves it, and in her flood of gratitude and thanks, she adds, "I wish you could make one of these for your own child."

"Gotcha."

❖ ❖ ❖

"Gotchas" lurk around every corner. They can be at the mall during your everyday shopping. Pregnant mothers and baby strollers with cute infants and toddlers host "gotchas" aplenty. "Gotchas" arise during holidays such as Christmas, Thanksgiving, Mother's and Father's Day. They show up at baseball games, during TV commercials, in comic strips, at company meetings.

Simply turn around, and there will probably be a reminder of your infertility. Whether or not it will affect you is often a matter of where you are at the moment in your walk with life. But, it is exactly at that moment when you most want to be in control of your life and emotions that out of the blue … a comment, a song, an object, or a memory … overwhelms you.

"Gotcha."

— Never Expect to be in Control —

Cat's in the Cradle

Ashley slept quietly in my lap as I waited at the doctor's office to have my ultrasound. She was a patient child. At four years of age, she had been through this many times since I started treatment when she was three.

Suffering from secondary infertility! What did that really mean? Formally, it meant I needed help from the medical community to get pregnant. But it meant so much more.

I could not live my life and one day find out I was pregnant. We conceived easily the first time and now we were going thorough all of these procedures and tests to conceive.

In one respect I was one of the more fortunate ones. I could stay home with my child. But these treatments took so much time and made me grumpy and tired.

At night, Ashley would want me to read to her, but I would be falling asleep, so she would take the book to her Dad. I couldn't tell her that I was tired because I wanted to have another child and the treatments were exhausting me. I was afraid she would think she was not good enough.

When she was two I would take her for long walks in the stroller around the neighborhood. Everyone would stop and talk with us. We don't walk anymore but sometimes when I drive by now they ask how Ashley is. I just smile and pretend that we are busy, when the reason we stopped walking is because it is too demanding on me.

At least she still takes a nap at four. None of my friends' children do. Maybe it is because we lie down together. Maybe she senses there is something wrong.

We've been here for forty-five minutes and the nurse still has not called my name. They must be busy today. I wish I could go home and put Ashley back to bed with me.

I often wonder if I am doing the right thing. Justin and I desperately want another child. A son would be nice. But are we neglecting Ashley? Should we not be satisfied with what we have and be glad we have more time to spend with Ashley since she is an only child?

Sometimes the doubts come crashing down. You spend so much time rushing off to some treatment that you feel you are neglecting your child.

When you have surgery, or need insemination, what do you do with the child? At times like this, I wish we lived in the same city as my relatives. It would be so much easier if I could drop off Ashley with her cousins. She could wake up in bed with them and they could play all morning. I could come back and have a cup of coffee with my sister before going home to start the rest of my day.

Oh, well, so much for dreaming. They just called my name. Poor Ashley, I must wake her again and for what? Maybe, just maybe, this time will work. I hope so — for Ashley's sake as well as ours.

— Oh, Those Holidays —

Can Holidays Be Holy?

A holiday is more than a day where you celebrate some special event or person. A holiday is steeped in tradition and passed from one generation to another. Holidays like Easter or Yom Kippur can define the very core of our belief systems. Holidays change the routine of life. Holidays are holy. Holidays are eternal. Holidays are tradition. You cannot pass traditions on to children you don't have. Where is eternity in just the two of you? What is holy about infertility?

Christmas and Hanukkah tend to be family gathering holidays, focusing on children as well as the event they commemorate. Similarly, holidays like Mother's Day and Father's Day honor parents who have children. On Mother's Day, you watch mothers receiving roses in church. On Father's Day, you miss having a child to participate with you in the three-legged race. On Easter, you watch other people's children search for eggs. On Christmas or Hanukkah, you watch children with happy faces opening their presents, while your dream of seeing your own child's happy face begins to die.

Holidays can provide a stark reminder to a couple of their infertility. Since many celebrations center on children, a couple feels they cannot fully participate because they do not have any. In seeing others enjoy themselves, they feel separate and left out, whether from their own actions or by being excluded.

They romanticize the celebrations into perfection. People ooh and aah over babies and young children. Stories are told of past family gatherings. Children do only good and cute things. Everyone has a wonderful time with no arguments of any kind.

Of course such romanticism is only a fantasy. But to an infertile couple, the focus of holidays on children emphasizes that they are not normal.

Certainly a couple can participate without children, and often do. Unfortunately, other family members may emphasize the feeling of being different by asking when the couple will have children. Or parents might remind them that more grandchildren would be nice.

And even if no one says anything, a couple tends to wonder. Why can't we have children? What is wrong with us? It is no wonder that the feelings of depression and negativity that a couple have held back tend to reassert during these gatherings.

An infertile couple's parents often have a hard time understanding why their children don't want to come over and open gifts with their siblings and their nieces and nephews. Or if they do come by, they don't understand why their grown children are in a bad mood. They spoil the whole holiday in their lack of participation! Parents ask why don't they just forget their troubles and enjoy the holiday/celebration along with everyone else.

Family gatherings can be even more difficult when others know you have been trying to start your family. Consolation and pity are often worse than silence.

Feeling separate and apart, feeling strange when trying to participate, and receiving consolation and pity only reminds you of what you don't have. No wonder holidays can be hard for an infertile couple.

You want to go to holiday gatherings because they are part of your heritage. You're glad to see that others have children; you wouldn't wish your infertility on them. On the other hand, you feel like you will spoil the party and are unable to participate, even if you try hard to forget your own problems.

You need to decide how you can best participate in holidays. Maybe you can visit after the presents are opened and there is less focus on the children and more on visiting and sharing a meal with family members. Maybe you can try to visit out of town family at times other than holidays when your emotions are less strained.

You need to find that compromise within yourself that allows you to both participate and maintain your own sense of well-being. You have relatives and will have relatives for the rest of your life, if you are

Acknowledging Your Emotions

fortunate. You don't want to be alone and adrift without family. But you need to decide what you can and cannot do during holiday periods.

Some couples participate fully. Others decide they can only visit family during non-holidays, when the focus is not on children. Some compromise by participating as much as they can, but avoid some particular holiday emotional hot spot.

Some people will not understand, or may even be jealous of you because of your freedom from children. Your decisions might seem extreme to them. For that there is no cure. You are dealing with the traditions of living and they affect everyone deeply. It is time to be strong and to protect both yourself and your spouse. There will come a time when your infertility issues are resolved. Maybe at that time you can change your decisions and once again fully participate in family holidays.

Notes

— Oh, Those Holidays —

We Won't Be Home for Christmas

I guess we grew up like most families in America where some holidays are traditionally spent with family. Sometimes family would consist of our own immediate family; sometimes it would include our extended family of grandparents, aunts, uncles, cousins, and/or maybe even close personal friends of my parents and their children.

Early in our marriage we expected a similar lifestyle. We would make sure that the little bit of vacation time we had was spent with one set of parents and generally our brothers would join us. Since Ryan and I are both first-born children, both sets of parents assumed that we would begin having their grandchildren first.

When Ryan's brother started his family, we enjoyed playing with our niece and nephew in anticipation that soon we would be ready to begin our family so our children could have cousins. However, our first child was still-born. We lost our second child early due to a miscarriage. Our plan to bring our niece and nephew some cousins was not going too well.

We continued to visit during holidays important to our parents, like Christmas and Thanksgiving, although I must admit that I missed our children during these celebrations. We had lots of hope that next year we would have a child or at least be pregnant. We did not envy Ryan's brother. We did, however, mourn our lack of children and wonder why we had to be broken.

Like most things, I guess, time is what finally changed our attitude. As one year after another passed and we remained childless, each holiday became more painful to share with our immediate families. We were continually reminded of the fact that we had no children to share in the holiday. By this time, my younger siblings were also beginning their families. My brother's wife had been pregnant when I was pregnant with our first child. So each holiday we spent with them we were not only reminded of our lack of children, but of the child we had lost.

At first the very idea that we would spend a major holiday away from one of our immediate families was difficult to accept. It was a long-standing tradition that we were reluctant to break. We struggled with the fact that we were more and more reluctant to visit during these major holidays. As time went on, we considered how painful it was to visit during each holiday and how much it had hurt us the year before. It wasn't as if we could just visit during Christmas afternoon, after all the presents were open. Not living close to either set of parents, a holiday visit was always a multi-day event.

We realized that when we visited during non-holiday times, we enjoyed our families much more and we did not mourn our own children in the same way. The fun we had was not because we were sharing the traditions of a holiday, but because we were taking time to do things together.

Finally, after a lot of grief and worry, we gave ourselves permission to become our own family. To us, this meant celebrating holidays with each other as a couple — not with our immediate families.

In announcing our plans to our families we were afraid that we would offend them. While we were gratified that offense wasn't taken, there was still a degree of hurt and a lack of understanding. We tried to explain, using the reasons you've just read, but they simply didn't make much sense to our families. "How come it's ok to visit in August, but not December? We're the same people in the summer as at Christmas …" To this day, they don't really understand why we do it, so we need to re-express our reasoning each year.

That reluctant acceptance didn't make our holidays more joyful. The idea of becoming our own family was scary. At first we were afraid that in trying to become a family of two, we would lose our dream of having children. Then we were afraid we would be lonely or homesick. As it turned out, it strengthened our dream of having our own children some day. The time alone during a major holiday gave us time to grow closer. Instead of sharing and giving to our families, we shared and gave to each other. We began to form traditions of our own that allowed us to uplift and comfort one another. Sometimes we would cry together, and sometimes we would rejoice. We began to rediscover why we were even taking the time to make this day special.

We now spend Christmas by ourselves and follow traditions we have begun, like our candle ceremony. On Christmas morning, we light a large unity candle to celebrate our uniting in marriage. Surrounding the unity candle are smaller candles, one candle for each anniversary of our marriage. We save the unity candle for burning long after Christmas to remind us of our love and how our marriage has endured through both good and painful times, like infertility.

Easter and Thanksgiving we spend in our home with friends we value and appreciate. Taking this time to honor our God and our friends, we've established traditions for these occasions as well. We serve lamb on Easter and gather around a large table for a formal dinner. We also have a "happiness check" to determine how our lives are progressing and determine if we want to change anything.

On Thanksgiving we usually do something different than the usual turkey. We love to cook so we find something unique to make where our friends can join in the preparation. These traditions are sometimes borrowed and sometimes new, but they help make what had become a chore to endure into a thankful and grateful day for us.

Nevertheless that doesn't make this a happy ending. Our families yearn to have us with them during these special times. And even though we've worked hard to come up with traditions to replace the familial times, we were still raised to look at holidays as family times. Ryan will often say, "It doesn't really feel like Christmas, does it?" And he'll be right. It's a Christmas we've made, rather than a Christmas we're used to.

In that sense, there is both a loss and a gain. The loss is in our families' lack of understanding of where we are during these times. The loss is in the fact that we wish with all our hearts that it could be different, that our children could be with us so that we could participate with them in happiness and harmony.

The gain is that we've done our best to appreciate and celebrate holy days with each other, because in the end, we are a family. It just happens to be a family of two.

— What We've Lost —

Can You Touch It?

Many people downgrade the loss of an infertile couple because they do not agree that they have lost anything. What an infertile couple has lost is the ability to bear children. This is a physiological, hormonal, and emotional loss that an infertile couple feels every day.

We talk about the freedom to choose our own destiny; to make our own free will choices. An infertile couple has lost their ability to choose to have children, a loss that greatly affects the destinies they may choose.

Others can decide whether and when to have children. An infertile couple cannot. Infertile couples have lost the chance to love and nurture a child from birth. Even if they eventually are able to have a child through birth or adoption, this loss of choice remains.

In understanding why this loss is a permanent scar, even if an infertile couple eventually succeeds in having children, we need to look at what society considers the phases of life:

We are born.
We go to school.
We get a job.
We get married.
We buy a house.
We have children.
We raise our children.
We retire.
We spoil our grandchildren.
We die.
Life goes on for our descendants.

When a person or couple can't take one of those basic steps, there is a loss. A loss must be grieved, whether openly or in secret. In this sense, the loss is not unique to the infertile couple.

Because most people live through the "phases of life" as stated above, they generally do not understand when you are not able to live them similarly.

Some people try to get you "back on track" in these phases of life. They can be quite blatant about their right to set you straight and get you to have children right now. For example, parents may ask where their grand children are. A friend or sibling says it is time you had the experience of getting up for midnight feedings like the rest of them. Others wisely keep their mouths quiet unless asked for their opinion.

Some people envy the fact that you are "off the track." They downplay an infertile couple's loss because they envy and resent the fact that the infertile couple has more time for different pursuits than child rearing. These people may also think that an infertile couple has more money, since it doesn't have to be spent on children. (In reality, treatment costs often eat up any "extra" money.)

Sometimes people who have children discount the loss of infertile couples as being unreal. They may say, "It is not as if you had a baby and it died." But to the infertile couple that is exactly how it feels.

And how do "we" feel about being "off the track"?

We miss what we expected. While we may have "freedom" from the "phases of life," it is a freedom we would trade in an instant for the shackles of parenthood.

What have we lost? All those things that we had looked forward to — our child's smile; cuddling at night; pillow fights; school plays starring our child; Little League or soccer games, we feel the loss constantly.

It is one thing to choose a different path, it is quite another to be forced to take a different road. By being forced to be "different" in the traditional phases of life, our feelings of loss and isolation can become paramount. The loss is not a baby whom we have literally held in our arms. The loss is the dream of having a child. The direction we desire for our life is out of reach and out of our control.

Acknowledging Your Emotions

Even if a pregnancy is finally achieved, infertility is a tremendous loss. It affects one's life profoundly. It leaves you with a sense of vulnerability. Like other major changes in life, it causes you to reevaluate everything you stand for and live for and to reexamine your hopes and dreams for the future.

The loss of children in your life can cause you to make drastic changes in the way you live your life. That is okay as long as the changes are not self-destructive. As with all life-affecting losses, the way to succeed is to move on, and to continue to try to do your best, even though you feel the loss every day.

Notes

— What We've Lost —

Can You See It?

I first became aware of how some people discount those who suffer from infertility at the weekly luncheon with my friends. To those who have children, it is as if infertility is not a problem or a loss, but rather good luck or a blessing. I know that everyone has problems, but when I tried to share mine, my friends only made me feel worse.

The day was particularly difficult for me because we had just finished our third cycle of ovary stimulation and my period had begun that morning. Jim and I were both devastated. We had been so hopeful that this time we would conceive the child we had been longing for. All morning I worked hard just to keep from crying.

On this luncheon date, everyone was in such a low mood that it became a pity party.

Doris has two sick parents, which is creating problems. She can't have them live with her since she is at work each day and can't provide the kind of care they need. Besides, they live in another city so it would mean a difficult move even if they did come to stay with Doris. None of her siblings live in the same city as her parents so they can't help either. She doesn't want to put her parents in a nursing home, but she doesn't know what else to do. Today she was particularly worried that she would have to use all of her vacation to settle this matter; what would her kids and husband say when they have no vacation this year?

Then Jennifer told us her husband had just been transferred to another city. She was devastated. She had just managed to get all her children into schools that she had personally interviewed! Now she was going to have to go through the same process again in a different city. The house they had been building was finally finished and they had only lived there three months. She just could not see spending time on all of these details again. In addition, it meant leaving her job! What was she going to do to earn a second paycheck if she did not find a job right away? And, she just could not bear to leave all of her friends, especially us. But, of course, the pay increase and added responsibility for Bob was going to be a great career move.

As Jennifer was finishing up, we heard Nancy softly crying. Nancy's daughter, Amanda, had not come home the night before and she had found evidence of her doing drugs. Amanda's counselor at school had been worried about her grades and performance in school, but was unaware of the drugs. Nancy did not even know where to start looking for Amanda. She had called the parents of the girls Amanda was friends with, but none of them knew anything about Amanda not coming home. Nancy did not know where to turn next. We all felt badly for Nancy, but none of us had any good advice for her.

I sat there listening to my friends and felt bad for all three of them. Then I started crying as well. Doris looked over at me and asked surprised, "Katie, what's wrong?" I just blurted out that I had started my period that morning. They looked dumbfounded until I broke down and told them that our third Pergonal cycle had not worked. When asked what Pergonal was, I found myself telling her that for the last two years Jim and I had been trying to have children. Pergonal was supposed to help me produce more eggs so I could hopefully get pregnant. I sounded so clinical to myself and started crying again. I told them that it was very depressing when such a personal and beautiful part of life, the creation of a child with your husband, was turned into a clinical process, monitored by infertility doctors.

I was the youngest of the group at twenty-eight years. Before today, I hadn't been sure if these women would understand what I was going through. After hearing them pour their hearts out over their problems, I just knew I could tell them. As I stopped crying, I began to notice the change in their faces. They looked at me in disbelief that not being pregnant could cause me pain. Jennifer said she was sorry I couldn't have children, but that I should be thankful I didn't have to go through the agony of finding the right school and neighborhood. It was a no win situation and she was so afraid that if she did not find the right school or the right neighborhood her children would end up as misfits.

Acknowledging Your Emotions

To make matters worse, Nancy blurted though tears that she wished her daughter had never been born. She could not understand why Amanda wanted to hurt her by doing drugs and staying out all night. She had raised her properly, gotten her into all the right schools, and given her the right toys and clothes. How could she do this to her? She told me to be grateful that I did not have to go through any of this, concluding that if she had to do it all over again, she wouldn't have had children.

Finally Doris spoke. She felt that if I wanted children, I should be able to have children, but reminded me that at least Jim and I had each other and were financially secure. She went on to say that when we finally had to face the problem of aging parents we would not have to worry about how we were going to pay for the arrangements and what to do with the children

I sat in stunned disbelief. I had just revealed a very personal and painful part of my life, and all my friends could say was to be grateful and feel lucky that I have free time, more money and a loving husband.

I felt so betrayed that I could not even begin to tell them of the strain this had put on our marriage. They could not understand that I had lost something.

Later I shared the story with my friend Linda, who was also going through infertility treatment. After talking it over, we decided that many people can't relate to us. They don't see or understand what we are going through. They don't know about the tests and the fertility drugs we take to try to get pregnant. They don't see how we have to schedule everything, even down to the time of intercourse. They don't understand the sorrow we go through since we have trouble even talking about it. They do not see our pain because they do not see anything physical we have lost.

To some, our unfulfilled dream of a family is not real. If you can't see it, you haven't lost it. Linda and I decided the loss of dreams could be just as real as a physical loss, and often, just as devastating, despite what others may decide for you.

Notes

Part 4
Dealing with Your Emotions

Sharing Your Pain with Others

    Cultivate Your Friends   151
    Security in Numbers   155

Handling What People Say

    What People Say   161
    Present Intense   169

Staying in Touch with Your Spouse

    Retreat with Your Spouse   173
    Betrayal and Healing   179

Dealing with Work

    When Work is in the Way   183
    "Dear Diary"   189

Accepting Others' Parenting Decisions

    You Can Do Better   197
    A Nightlight for Her Worries   199

Giving Love to Pets

    Pets as Therapy   201
    Knight in Shining Armor   203

Quote on page 151 is from a speech
by Janet L. Lazo-Davis in 1990.

— Sharing Your Pain with Others —

Cultivate Your Friends

"Your pain is always the worst" — *and the happiest situation is always either of your own making or from your acceptance of the things that will make you happy. The most painful situation is always your own. So is the potential for the happiest.*

There is a commonly held belief that we can't understand others' pain unless we have been through the same situation.

When we have lost something of great importance, we often feel that no one else has pain worse than ours. As a result, others can't understand! They have not experienced our pain, and therefore could not hurt as much.

When you are willing to admit and talk about your problem, it seems that others with the same or similar problem come out of the woodwork. This is also true with infertility problems — many people experiencing infertility do not talk about the subject except to those who share the same problem.

Given the commonly held belief that only those who have your problem can understand you, it is helpful to share your pain. That is why help groups like RESOLVE are so useful. Shared adversity is a bonding that often ends up transcending the adversity itself.

We encourage you to take advantage of sharing with those who can truly understand and feel your pain. Pain always seems to lessen in doing this, whether the pain is infertility or anything else. But does that mean the belief is true: that the only people who can understand your pain are those who have gone through it?

We'll be the first to agree that it is *easier* to understand your pain if we've been through it ourselves. Having gone through infertility, we are much more capable of understanding and empathizing than if we had not.

However, most of us have suffered a major loss or tragedy in our lives, and therefore experienced strong emotions of grief and anger that come with severe pain.

Such losses may not help others better understand why an infertile person hurts, but it can allow them to accept that an infertile couple does experience pain and distress. In other words, a sympathetic person can translate his/her remembrance of pain into a semblance of yours and thus can be understanding of your pain.

Simply having someone acknowledge that your pain and loss is genuine can help. The problem with infertility is that many people do not agree that you have lost anything. Many will focus more on what you have rather than what you have lost. Your pain is not visible to many. They do not see that the struggle to have a child is fundamental to the core of your being and that you will hurt for a long time, probably for the rest of your life. They do not see that the loss of a dream or the loss of hope can be as painful as any other kind of major loss.

For those who are wrapped up in their own little world, do not be surprised when they do not translate their pain in a different area into a way to be sympathetic to your pain. It is very likely that they are not sympathetic to others in general, although seeing pain often forces them to acknowledge it in some fashion. It is simply easier to dismiss your pain when they cannot see it.

Consider yourself richer when you find friends who accept your loss and make you feel accepted in spite of your loss. They may not have ever had any problems conceiving their children, but they can see that you hurt because you do. They don't dismiss, accuse or blame. They do not feel that you did something wrong to deserve this. If you share in their children's lives, they do not flaunt them as if they have a prize and you do not. They also know the only words of comfort are: "I am sorry. I realize it is painful for you."

Dealing with Your Emotions

Handling pain, we have found, is a three-step process.

1. Acknowledge your pain rather than shutting it up deep inside you where it will fester.

2. Express your pain. Expressing it to someone who has gone through the same pain is usually the easier path, because they will probably be able to empathize (although some people won't empathize even then).

3. Move on from the pain. This process often takes the most time.

Pain doesn't discriminate based on the cause. Your pain is always the worst because it is the ***pain you feel*** rather than the pain you understand is in others. Understanding that allows you to deal with your own pain as well as help others deal with theirs.

Notes

— Sharing Your Pain with Others —

Security in Numbers

RESOLVE meetings and socials can be a very healthy experience for infertile couples. They are sometimes the only place where people feel comfortable talking about the loss of their fertility. They can be informative about current treatments and which physicians are performing them. You can also make connections with other people experiencing infertility that could lead you to much needed support. We highly recommend exploring this avenue early on in your struggle with infertility.

The following anecdote is about a RESOLVE social. All the characters and their stories are fictional representations. The material presented here is based on interviews with willing infertile couples. It did not come from RESOLVE meetings or socials, as those meetings are considered confidential.

✧ ✧ ✧

Susan was thrilled at the large turnout. There were twenty women in her living room waiting for the social to begin. As she looked around at the faces, she saw some very dear friends and quite a few new visitors with looks of anticipation.

Susan was determined that newcomers would feel as welcome as she had been made to feel when she attended her first RESOLVE social. The pain of trying to have a child was bad enough. At least by banding together in support of one another, they might reduce some of the pain of infertility.

Jennifer was prepared to do a program on the cost of treatments and insurance reform. However, Susan felt that since there were a lot of visitors an "everyone tells their story" format might allow the newcomers some stress relief.

She liked to use this format whenever there were enough new stories to make the evening unique. In addition to helping others, she found the new visitors' stories to be helpful to herself by seeing how far she had come over the years in dealing with her own pain.

She was thankful that her healing was so far along, and credited RESOLVE in helping her accept her infertility. There were very few outside of RESOLVE whom she could talk to about the pain she had gone through.

As the hostess, Susan started the meeting, welcoming everyone and explaining a little about RESOLVE and how its purpose was to help infertile couples. She also reminded participants not to mention medical doctors by name in the meeting. RESOLVE did not endorse or criticize anyone in the medical profession. If anyone wanted to discuss their personal medical counsel, they could do so privately. She explained the format of the meeting of each sharing their stories and then proceeded to tell her own story.

In the meantime Michelle sat uncomfortably in her chair. Dreading her turn, she kept counting the number of people who would go before her and wondered if she could tell these women (and one man!) her story. It was so painful. Because of these feelings she could only half listen to Susan discussing how she and her husband Jeremy found out they were infertile.

However, Michelle was encouraged when she heard that Susan had originally been scared about finding the wrong doctor, but ended up with a doctor who truly cared and who was so proficient that she discovered her and Jeremy's problem in the first six months. Michelle didn't understand much about the problem itself, but at least it sounded as if Susan may have gone through some of the things she herself had been experiencing. But, since Susan and Jeremy's problem didn't seem to match what Michelle felt she and Rick were going through, her attention turned to the woman after Susan. Jennifer was so stunningly beautiful that she reminded Michelle of a young movie star. How could stunningly beautiful women be infertile? They are the epitome of how you strive to look! How could anything be wrong in her life? As Michelle listened to Jennifer, she began to grieve for her. Jennifer had severely misshapen fallopian tubes, so the only way she could possibly conceive was through in vitro fertilization. What a terrible thing to learn! Michelle was not even sure if she and Rick would consider high tech. Michelle crossed her fingers and hoped it would not take much longer for her or Jennifer to have children.

Heather and Caroline were next in line to tell their respective stories. Their stories were similar in that they had each lost a child in the fourth month of their pregnancy.

Michelle got tears in her eyes as Heather related how she had held her four-month pre-term child in her arms in the hospital. The doctor had suggested they name the child and have a funeral. Heather said she regretted having a miscarriage, but counted her blessings that the child had died from a rare birth defect that was not genetic and therefore probably would not reappear in another pregnancy. Heather concluded by saying that although they were having trouble getting pregnant again, the doctor was optimistic that they would soon conceive.

When it was Caroline's turn, she couldn't start, because she was crying. Heather reached over to hold her, and soon Caroline calmed down enough to tell everyone that she had also lost her child in the fourth month of pregnancy. It still hurt her to talk about the ordeal. What if the next child also died? Through her tears she explained that she did not always cry when she talked about trying to get pregnant. It was just that she was taking Clomid and it made her very emotional.

Michelle wondered why it was easier for Heather to tell her story than Caroline. How did Heather accept the pain that Caroline had not been able to?

Suddenly it was her turn. Michelle blurted out, "How do you make the pain go away?" While the rest of the women were silent, Susan in a quiet but factual voice said, "The pain never goes away. Over the years it may lessen, but it never goes away. The longer you deal with the mental and emotional pain, the more you have to learn to appreciate what you do have. You need to begin to release the anger and to accept that in your life, the trial to begin a family is something you must deal with. When frustration sets, in you need a friend who can listen and who cares." Susan then asked, "Would you like to tell us of your journey into the realm of infertility, Michelle?"

Stunned, Michelle just sat there thinking, "Susan remembered my name, and I'd only told it to her once." She cares! This thought helped Michelle loosen up as she told how she and Rick found out that she had anti-sperm antibodies, and therefore were not able to get pregnant the usual way, but had to resort to IUI. They were both scared to mention this to their parents, since both sets really wanted grandchildren. None had been born yet, and since they were both the oldest, it was somehow their obligation to have the first grandchildren. Michelle heard the anguish and frustration in her own voice. "Everyone makes getting pregnant sound so easy. One month you decide and the next month it happens!"

The woman next to Michelle agreed. Melody related that when her sister was in law school and decided to have children, she figured out when it would be most convenient to give birth and then calculated backwards to determine which month she should conceive so as not to hamper her law school schedule. Like clockwork, she got pregnant.

The frustration of hearing her sister telling this story was too much for Melody to bear. She had stopped going to some family gatherings because her sister would chide her about waiting so long to start a family, valuing her career over children. Her sister would say things like, "Children really could be so charming! They aren't that hard to take care of. Don't you even want children?"

Realizing that Melody was getting agitated, Michelle patted her hand. Melody then told the group how endometriosis was causing her pain, and was the reason why she could not conceive. She regretted the fact that she and her husband had waited so long to start. If only they had realized that fertility was not something you could always control, they would have started sooner.

When Bonnie's turn came, she asked those in the group who were on Pergonal to raise their hands, and then asked everyone to sign a petition to go to the insurance commissioners to try to get health care coverage for couples on high-tech infertility treatments. Given the fact that currently employers could choose whether or not to pay for infertility coverage, the petition requested that infertility be defined as

Dealing with Your Emotions

a disease which would then have to be covered. Michelle was stunned to realize that someone had put that much work into a petition. Were the medical costs that high? She hoped that she and Rick were pregnant soon, as she wasn't sure they could afford these kinds of costs.

Rita spoke next. It seemed that Rita had undiagnosed infertility. The doctors seemed at a loss as to what was not working correctly. She explained what treatment the doctor was trying and asked if anyone had gone through the same. Several had been through the same treatments and made a few suggestions that might help.

As Michelle sat through the rest of the social, Susan watched her visibly relax. Jeremy, who had tried to stay in the background all evening, told his wife that her intuition had been right. Michelle was definitely one who needed to get out some of the confusion, anger and frustration that she was feeling. Susan was thankful that it was turning out to be a good program.

After everyone had left, Susan and Jennifer talked about the social. They realized they had come a long way in their emotional state as compared to their first RESOLVE function. There were still major issues in their infertility journey, but they were able to see blessings they could count.

Notes

— Handling What People Say —

What People Say

People say the strangest things, especially when they are uncomfortable, confused or embarrassed. Unfortunately, this includes rude, insensitive, and thoughtless comments. This is true in any situation.

Many people are embarrassed about your infertility, especially if they are not infertile themselves. Wanting to dismiss the topic to get back to more comfortable ground, they end up making a flippant or a dismissive remark, or a joke.

Many do not consider your infertility a serious, permanent, or life-changing problem. If you told them you had cancer, that you were dealing with a parent with Alzheimer's, or that your child was spaced out on drugs, their response would often be much more serious. They would still be uncomfortable, but in all likelihood would make a more fervent attempt to say something compassionate before trying to change the subject.

Even if they do give your infertility some credence, many joke about it. Unlike disease, death, or similar tragedies, there are no pat responses to the revelation that you are infertile. Emotions are close together. People may laugh at funerals meaning to cry. Thus, you may get an uncomfortable joking response even from someone who truly cares.

In most cases when insensitive remarks are made, the best course of action is to ignore them as much as possible. Any repartee will usually be taken negatively. As a result, you will probably end up being seen as oversensitive or rude yourself, even if you are totally justified in your reply. People who make these kinds of remarks usually do so without thinking. Thus, they will probably not think through your reply either, so your response won't do any good.

It's hard not to release your wrath, given you have heard the same remark from others time and again. Here are some of them; we're pretty sure you've heard them all.

"Just relax, you'll get pregnant!"

This is probably the most popular, often well-meant, but infuriating statement made to someone trying to get pregnant. It implies that you are doing something wrong. You not only can't get pregnant, but you're stressed out about it. Being stressed is the real reason you aren't pregnant.

Why do some people believe this? Well, usually, they had no trouble getting pregnant themselves. Their pregnancy may have resulted suddenly without warning. In other words, it happened "just like that," during a time when they were not worrying about it. So, for many people, pregnancy occurs when one is *not* thinking about it, making it very easy to pass on this feeling to someone who is obviously worrying "overmuch" about pregnancy. If you'd just quit worrying about it so much, it would happen.

This response totally dismisses (and probably never even considers) medical conditions such as hormonal issues, male sterility, infrequent ovulation, inability to carry to term, and the myriad other reasons one cannot get pregnant.

This statement is the equivalent of, "Hey, just relax, and the cancer will go away!" But since no one believes that cancer will go away, no one makes such a remark. People do believe, however, that infertility is a thing that will just go away. It went away for them when they became pregnant, right?

Belief in this statement is infuriating because these "true believers" are not only saying that your problem is within you by not relaxing, but that your real medical problem is not the primary issue, so you are doubly wrong in how you are acting in trying to get pregnant.

My number one comeback to these people (no, in our society, you aren't allowed to punch them in the nose ...) is to disarm them by agreeing with them on one point. My response is usually, "Ok, you're right. There is one way that stress prevents a couple from getting pregnant. If stress causes a couple to have less sex, then the likelihood of them getting pregnant is less."

This statement still dismisses the complex facts that probably surround any infertile couple. Many can't get pregnant by "just having sex," and many end up increasing their stress by having to time when they have sex. But the response usually casually disarms insistent well wishers who stick to their insulting, but often well-meant belief.

One final take on this: For a small minority of couples, the statement is actually true. Stress does cause strange problems, and infertility just might be one result. But for the vast majority where it is not true, the statement just does not hold, and should not be made.

"If you adopt, you'll get pregnant. It happens all the time."

In one sense, this statement is a direct corollary to "Just relax, you'll get pregnant." Since you don't seem to be able to relax and get pregnant, all you need to do is adopt. Since you have a kid, you'll stop worrying about getting pregnant and **boom**, you'll get pregnant because you finally stopped worrying about it.

This belief is adhered to by even more people than the "just relax" statement because they have documented evidence to prove it.

Their cousin's friend adopted, and then got pregnant. So did their lawyer's daughter. And unlike urban legends for which you can never find the documented proof, they can walk you right up to the lawyer's daughter who will proudly announce that "Yes indeed we did" adopt, and then later got pregnant.

Case closed. Go out; adopt a child, and suddenly your infertility worries will be over.

In reality, the probability that you will get pregnant after adopting is the same as getting pregnant before adopting. But when someone with infertility problems adopts and then gets pregnant, it is news. News changes people's perception of probability. Planes seem to crash all the time if you watch the headlines. The headlines don't announce how many times all of the other planes landed safely.

So, although people can indeed point out friends who adopted and then got pregnant, you could find the same percentage of people who didn't adopt and then got pregnant. Unfortunately, the former group is much more visible, because everyone talks about it.

"You can have mine!"

A joke! How funny. They're trying to dismiss your problem by pretending that having children is an awful experience. Of course they are not really willing to give up their children, nor would you take them. The statement ends up being infuriating because all it does is emphasize the fact that they have children when you do not.

"Oh, I am fertile Myrtle!"

Why do people think that by showing how they are the opposite of you they are helping you out?

"If you'd only ... do whatever is popular at the moment ... you'd get pregnant."

This is an attempt to give advice and be sympathetic, but it ends up coming across as an authoritative statement. It implies that you aren't giving your situation enough thought.

"You'll get pregnant next month ..."

This is another dismissive statement. The person wants to move away from the topic by implying the problem will go away soon.

"Take a vacation and you'll get pregnant."

This is a variant on the "Just relax" response. It would be nice if it were true.

"You're lucky. Look at all the freedom and extra money you have!"

This is an attempt to turn your "problem" into an advantage. It is not only dismissive; it denies you have a problem. It further implies that you are blessed rather than in pain. It is extremely insulting. Unfortunately, it is often the people who come close to understanding your problem who make it. They have thought about your situation and are trying to be optimistic and positive. Unfortunately, their conclusion is often totally erroneous. They haven't seen your tight medical schedule or your sky-rocketing doctor's bills.

"Kids are such a pain!"

At least the people making this remark aren't offering you their own. This is another dismissive statement implying that you are better off not even pursuing pregnancy.

And so on ...

I'm sure you can think of many more remarks of this kind. The bottom line is that you will hear many. We recommend that your response be to remain silent and move on; which is what the people making these ill-considered statements should have done in the first place:

What Is the Correct Thing to Say?

Now that we've dealt with all of the insensitive things that people may say, well-meaning or otherwise, let's remember that not everyone makes such remarks. Many people do think the issue through and respond appropriately and sensitively.

A friend of mine is the mother of several children. She had no problems getting pregnant, but her heart went out to us because we could not share the same joys. She asked me, "What do you say to a couple who are having problems having children?" I told her that she had already taken the proper first step, and that "the best thing you can do is to simply acknowledge our pain and loss. Don't feel pity for us, but realize that we hurt and that we have a right to hurt. We have been denied something that is a vital part of our being, the right to bear children. Initially, I never questioned whether I had control over my fertility, so realizing that I didn't came as a shock."

"You've accepted that I am struggling without being uncomfortable or embarrassed by my struggling. You allow me to feel my loss. You agree

I have lost something, but you don't pity me. You don't flaunt your healthy children or make me feel guilty by saying that I would have children if I had done things differently."

"You don't discount my feelings by saying things like 'you can have mine'. You are willing to share your children, but you don't apologize for being able to have children. You realize you are blessed with children, but you don't take them for granted. You don't make me feel different for not having any."

"You don't feel sorry for me, but you provide sympathy. You accept that I am worth something even if I haven't been able to give birth and raise children of my own."

"Some people make me feel worthless since I can't produce children. You make it clear that my worth is not based on how many children I have. My worth is in my actions and deeds, not in my childbearing ability."

"When I am depressed about not having children, I can talk with you and you listen without being judgmental. You lovingly accept my hurt and help me through the healing process. You didn't laugh when I told you I was going to try to write a book on infertility. You encouraged me even when my first attempts at writing weren't very polished."

"You realize I am grieving for something that can not be seen or touched. You support me as I go through medical treatments. You understand I am seeking a new purpose in life, because I thought my purpose was to have and raise children. You offer me a shoulder to cry on as I begin to explore the what-ifs of never having children or the what-ifs of adoption."

"You know that even if I have a child, a lot of my innocence will still have been lost and the pain of the effort to have that child will still be there."

"To be succinct, you are my friend."

Understanding friends have helped us through trying emotional times by allowing us to grieve. When she brought over a list asking for critique, I asked if we could use it in this section of our book. She was pleased.

Here is her summary:

1. Realize that the only consolation you can give is to be willing to listen.

2. Listen without criticism and judgment. You may not agree with some of the choices they make or have made, but these burdens and decisions are not yours. You don't have to live daily with the consequences of their decisions.

3. Let them know they are loved and accepted for who they are. Their reproductive ability is not a measure of their worth.

4. Acknowledge their pain and their loss.

5. Allow them to grieve for the children they may never have or for those lost to miscarriage or early delivery.

6. Only offer an opinion when it is asked for. Do not second guess their choice of treatment or doctor.

7. Be as positive and uplifting as you can. However, do not say, "I just know you will get pregnant." What will you say if they don't get pregnant?

8. Don't be embarrassed by some of the things you hear. Fertility involves sex.

9. Realize that the only real comfort to an infertile couple is succeeding in having a child of their own, whether through birth or adoption. Judgmental comments on either their efforts or final decision in this matter will not help.

10. Realize that this is a difficult time in their life. Simply care about them. That goes a long way toward understanding their plight.

Notes

— Handling What People Say —

Present Intense

Dale and I were excited. We were going to our ten-year high school reunion and had not seen many of our classmates since we graduated. Both of us had gone away to college, and after we married, we took jobs in another state. We were looking forward to seeing everyone. There was so much catching up to do.

The before-dinner conversation was mostly "remember when" types of things, like the class picnic where everyone got poison ivy. Dinner went smoothly, but when it came to the after-dinner conversation, we soon felt like total outsiders.

Somehow the conversation focused on who had married whom and how many kids they had. I guess it was the funny award ceremony that started it by announcing how many were married before twenty and who had the most kids, but the conversation around our table continued to stay on children and schools and other children-type things. Whenever we were asked about our kids, we'd shrug and say that the time was not right yet. We couldn't reveal how we had tried for the last three years and had not been able to get pregnant.

The whole conversation was alien to us. We both were career people, and fairly proud of our jobs. At the moment, we were only hearing conversations about people's problems with their children, involving day care, formula, and teachers. I probably would have been complaining with the rest of them if I had been in their shoes, but all I could think about was, "Why couldn't they talk positively about something rather than saying kids are a pain and here is all the trouble they cause?"

We tried to start up conversations about jobs and careers; occasionally we even succeeded for a time.

All evening, I tried to find Marcie. She and I were best friends in high school and we had lost touch. Finally I spotted Judy who had also hung around with Marcie and me, so I asked her where Marcie was. She said that Marcie had four children and had not been able to get a baby sitter, but was looking forward to the picnic the next day. She was glad the committee had decided on a picnic so we could bring our children. Judy and I chatted about our days in school together and then shared facts about our current lives that were so different. She spent her days at home with her two children, ages two and five, while I was a career woman. She seemed very interested in what I told her about my job repeating several times that she wished she had finished college. I did not think much about it then, but later it hit me that she envied how I was able to have a career.

At our hotel later that evening, Dale and I discussed whether we wanted to go to the picnic. Having been regaled with tales about our friends' children, we worried that it might be worse the next day with all the children present, but after a good night's sleep we decided to go. Besides, I would see Marcie.

Whereas the dinner was formal and elegant, the picnic was rowdy. Nothing seemed organized. I finally found Marcie and breathed a sigh of relief — we could talk and maybe the picnic would be saved. As I got closer, and she recognized me, she called out, "Where are your children?" Two of her four were at her feet and the others were close by. I told her the usual story about how we were not ready for children yet and the conversation went down hill from there. She started to lecture me on how you had to get started so you could have grand children before you were too old, etc. I wanted to tell her to shut up, to yell, "You've changed. You don't know!" But that was the point. She didn't know. I couldn't fault her for talking like she did based on what I had told her.

As soon as I found Dale in the crowd, I told Marcie I needed to go. But before we could make our escape, we ran into another friend and his wife whom we had been close to in high school. They had brought their two children. Finally, the dreaded question came up about us not having any children with us at the picnic. Ignoring our normal response, they asked if we were experiencing trouble having children. Surprised, we hesitantly said yes. They laughed, and told us not to worry, because we'd get pregnant soon. In the mean-time, they offered one of theirs!

I realized later that no one knew what to say to us. A lot of it was our own fault, because we didn't explain what our situation was. They simply wanted to share their current lives with us, whereas all we wanted to do was to remember the past because we didn't want to review our present childless state. The only common ground came when we managed to talk about jobs and careers; but, for most people, that was only half of the conversation to be shared.

We should have arrived with a thicker skin. We couldn't expect people to be sympathetic when they didn't know what to be sympathetic about. We should have known what we were getting into. We'll know better next time.

Notes

— Staying in Touch with Your Spouse —

Retreat with your Spouse

As we walk on our path through life and infertility, we sometimes focus on certain parts to the exclusion of others. As a result, we can end up ignoring, neglecting or taking for granted something we cherish. Often, this includes our spouse. We get so focused on having a child that we lose focus on the person who is right there with us.

With treatments, work, activities, chores, and all the other things that take up time in your life, there never seems to be the time or the right words to discuss with your spouse the fears, the frustration and the hopes of the infertility process. It is easy to ignore the subject except for going through the motions suggested by the doctor. Communication is fragile at best. It is hard to know what another person is thinking and feeling because you have only your own reactions and experiences to compare it to. Your spouse may not have a similar framework to explain his or her feelings in a way that allows you to understand. Unfortunately, the end result can sometimes be separation or divorce.

In addition to the pitfalls of communication in general, men and women react differently to problems. Women often want to talk about problems, whereas men often want to ignore them, push them aside, or pretend they don't exist. These different reactions to the same situation can exacerbate the lack of communication that might be occurring.

Sometimes, simply understanding these general differences can lead to improved communication. For example, knowing that your husband doesn't want to talk about infertility, can lead to a loving statement like the following, "I know you don't want to talk about this right now, but I need to talk about it some time. When can we talk? You decide — tell me when you can listen."

You need to gain a mutual understanding of where both parties are coming from in order to avoid becoming isolated from each other. Given our busy everyday lives, you need to schedule enough time to talk. If you can do it piecemeal, that's fine. But often, it takes a weekend or more of devoted time to achieve an adequate level of communication.

A retreat with your spouse may be a great solution. Don't try to do a retreat at home, as you will find too many reasons to interrupt your conversation. You can go on an organized retreat or create one of your own.

There are many organized ways to have a personal retreat. Some recommend the model of "Marriage Encounter" groups, designed to help spouses get to know what each other is thinking and feeling. Once you know how to communicate with your spouse and have practiced it, it becomes easier. Discussions of important issues become easier because you have done the painful part of learning how to talk and more importantly how to listen. You also learn to respect your spouse more.

If you prefer to create your own retreat, we have compiled a few guidelines for a successful retreat. These guidelines helped us, but we encourage you to be creative and modify them to suit your own needs. The goal is to end up with a more open relationship with your spouse and reaffirm that you are a family. If you've been growing apart, you will hopefully begin to come closer to one another again through this process.

We have divided the retreat guidelines into two parts. The first is for those who have limited time. The second is for those who can take a time to relax in conjunction with a retreat.

Guidelines for a Personal Spouse Retreat

Prepare ahead of time for the retreat by focusing on the issues you will bring to the discussion. Realize that you and your spouse may be at different stages of understanding where your issues reside. It is very destructive to blame your spouse for what is happening, and no healing will occur as a result of this type of discussion. If there are issues where healing and forgiveness need to be given for past actions, it might be helpful to seek professional counseling.

Realize that this is your life partner. When you married, you wanted to make this person your partner in life with love in mind. Now make the choice to make your spouse your partner with both love and respect. You can be there for each other.

Remember that your own needs must be met before you can begin to help someone else meet his or hers. Sometimes a retreat is needed to just define what your needs are. A second retreat can be scheduled to discuss a plan for meeting those needs. Taking time between the retreats will help you sort out your feelings about each other's needs.

Before you go on the retreat, prepare in your mind or on paper a list of expectations to share with your spouse, and set goals to be accomplished by the end of the retreat.

Take time to empty your mind of all other things (like work schedules) so the retreat will be successful. Catch up on sleep if you need to. Sometimes you need to meet your body needs before you can be compassionate with someone else. Finally, don't try to conquer anything. Allow yourselves to relax between discussions.

A Weekend Retreat

Here are the basics. In preparation you may wish to come up with initial answers to the following questions. It will improve the weekend you take for this retreat. Obviously, we are focusing on infertility; you may wish to add other topics.

1. Discuss Goals for Infertility Treatment:

    ❖ How important is it to each of us to have children?

    ❖ What high-tech treatments are we willing to pursue?

    ❖ How many treatments will we pursue before we reevaluate?

    ❖ When will we seek another medical opinion if things are not working?

    ❖ If the treatments fail, what are our options?

    ❖ How do we feel about adoption?

    ❖ Are we at a point where we should start discussing living childfree?

2. Discuss Expectations of One Another:

    ❖ How should we compromise on important issues where we disagree?

    ❖ Are we properly allocating work and chores?

    ❖ Are we making enough time for each other? To have fun? To enjoy life?

    ❖ Are there activities in our lives we need to say 'No!' to at this point?

A Longer Retreat

If you can schedule a week or more, add the following:

Make this a mini-vacation, but don't forget the retreat. Add a couple of favorite things to do and share. Pick things to do where you can renew the closeness you shared in your relationship before things got so hectic: like walking, listening to music, watching a fire, or having a nice dinner together.

Make time for intimate sharing as well, in a relaxed and unpretentious fashion. The goal here is to enjoy one another as you used to without having to focus on whether this will be the time you conceive.

✧ ✧ ✧

By taking time to grow close again, you will find that you will be able sort out your feelings about the infertility issues you face. Maybe you will also find that you have made some incorrect assumptions about what your spouse was feeling and thinking.

After a retreat where you can open your heart to your spouse, you may begin to make the changes that are necessary for your lives to improve. Maybe it will simply involve complimenting each other more. Maybe it will be taking time to hear the fears you are encountering during the treatments. It is often the simplest changes that have the most value.

Whatever the changes necessary, they should help you be more sensitive to your spouse's needs and result in a more relaxing environment during an otherwise stressful time. You need all the allies you can get in dealing with infertility. Make sure your spouse is one!

Notes

— Staying in Touch with Your Spouse —

Betrayal and Healing

Bill and Denise see me once a week for counseling. They have been infertile for three years, which has caused some marital problems. They came to me after Bill had an extramarital affair, hoping I could help them heal and that in the process their marriage would be saved. Before that could happen, however, they had to learn how to communicate with one another.

For quite some time, Bill and Denise had been seeing a specialist who had recommended the routine procedures to correct the problems they had with conception. During this process, Bill found himself drawn to women, who were fertile; in particular, a divorced lonely woman with three children who worked for him.

Denise fell apart when she found out about the affair and was the one who insisted the two of them get some counseling. Bill reluctantly agreed. It was their infertility specialist who referred them to me.

When I come into the picture late in a situation such as this, the first question I ask is, "Do you want to save your marriage?" Unless both partners are willing to work with one another, they will not be able to save the relationship. I was pleased to see that both Bill and Denise wanted to save their marriage.

In our last session I felt Bill and Denise would be able to heal their marriage. It would be painful, but they both appeared to want to trust one another again.

✧ ✧ ✧

Counselor: "Bill, can you explain to Denise why you had an affair?"

Bill: "Lately, when Denise and I make love, all we are doing is trying to make a baby. Our lovemaking is no longer satisfying. It is so scheduled, so routine. Denise only seems to want to make love when she is fertile, and then we must always do "this" or "that" to get the desired results. It is no longer enjoyable. We've lost all spontaneity and passion. When I was with Beth I felt virile and wanted. For *me*, not just for my sperm."

Denise: "I didn't know you felt that way!"

Counselor: "Bill, what did you hope to accomplish with your affair, did you hope to get the woman pregnant?"

Bill: "Absolutely not! Well … maybe I did. I did not really want her pregnant when I thought about it, but she found me so desirable that I did not want to resist. I felt virile when we made love. She was so lonely since her husband left her. After all, she had three children. I knew she was fertile and maybe I wanted to prove that I was also. Maybe secretly I felt that if she did conceive I would prove something."

Counselor: "Does that mean that Denise is less of a woman since she had not been able to have children?"

Bill: "No! In fact when I started thinking what I had done and how it was wrong, I felt ashamed. I was ruining the relationship I had with Denise. I was killing our love. I wasn't really in love with this other woman. I did not want to be married to her. Denise is my life partner. I guess I just wanted to feel that I was a virile man. Sex with Beth helped me to do that."

Counselor: "Does this mean that when you and Denise make love you don't feel like a man?"

Bill: "Well, most of the time when we make love we must do all of those things to get pregnant. I must admit that I feel like a machine, not a man. And I don't feel virile. After all, we're not having kids, are we?"

Counselor: "Denise, what do you feel when you make love with Bill?"

Denise: "That maybe I will get pregnant this month. That if I get pregnant, all of the treatment will have been worth it. I didn't realize Bill felt like a machine. I thought he wanted children as much as I did."

Counselor: "How much do the two of you talk to one another about the treatments you are going through and what you each feel about it?"

Denise: "We talk a lot about the things the doctor says we must do, but we don't seem to talk much about how if affects us in general. I guess we both just want to have a baby and get on with our lives. We sort of feel our lives are on hold right now."

Bill: "I'm just trying to have kids because Denise wants them so much. I guess I want them, too, or else I wouldn't need to feel virile. But we just go through what the doctor says to do each month and that is about it. We don't seem to talk much any more. Denise seems to be too tired to do anything, and when her period starts she is really depressed."

Counselor: "Denise, do you feel abandoned by Bill?"

Denise: "I feel mostly I am a failure and not attractive anymore."

Counselor: "Do you feel that Bill still loves you and wants to stay married to you?"

Denise: "I don't know."

Counselor: "Bill, are you still attracted to Denise? And, if yes, why?"

Bill: "I love Denise very much. I think she is a good wife and would make a wonderful mother. I am sorry that she has not been able to have children yet for both our sakes, but I know that I would be lost without all of the little things she does for me."

Counselor: "Bill, do you think you will ever be tempted to have an affair again?"

Bill: "I don't know. That's the reason I agreed to come to a counselor. I want to know how to avoid it in the future. I figured that the only way I could save my marriage would be to get some help in talking about all of the problems we haven't talked about in the past. Mostly we need to talk about this stupid problem of not being able to have kids."

✧ ✧ ✧

The three of us continued to talk for the rest of their hour. It was obvious Bill and Denise needed to learn to talk about their feelings. I could help them there, but they also had to learn to talk to one another day to day about any future problems as they arose.

After this session I hope they learned that problems don't just go away. They can be faced together if they discuss them and listen carefully to each other.

— Dealing with Work —

When Work Is in the Way

Work is something we can't ignore. It's what we do every day to earn a living. These days, work is a fact of life for both the man and woman; even when one of the two does stay home, there are often day to day activities equivalent to work.

In regards to infertility, the issue with work is that you end up dealing with the same group of people day in and day out. You have to make decisions on how to interact with them professionally, socially, and emotionally.

Marriages, sicknesses in the family, deaths, and births are all "events" in the workplace. Even if you work for a large company, you tend to also work for a subgroup in that company that reacts to these events.

Because of this, you must be able to react appropriately when such events arise. If someone has died, you are expected to help comfort. If someone is being married, you are expected to help congratulate. And if someone is giving birth, you are expected to rejoice.

This isn't always easy. If you are recently divorced, it can be hard to be congratulatory of a new marriage. If you recently had a death in the family, it is hard to rejoice at someone else giving birth. Luckily, our social structure allows such excuses. As long as people are aware that you are having a difficult time, it behooves them to excuse your lack of participation due to your circumstance.

Unfortunately, not getting pregnant is not readily recognized as a legitimate excuse. I'm not saying this is universally true; in some environments, that is also a valid excuse from recognizing painful events, and hopefully is becoming more recognized as valid.

The issue is the work environment where infertility is not recognized as a legitimate reason for staying aloof from celebratory events, especially other women's pregnancies.

How can you get excited about a woman's second or third child when you are trying desperately to have one? The answer is that you can't. We're not saying that you can't participate, put on a happy face, and in fact be genuinely happy for the expectant mother. Some people have that ability, even during their own issues with infertility. For those who can do that, we admire their fortitude.

However, excitement is probably not the correct term even for those blessed people who can look past their own problems. For most of us, dread would be more appropriate.

It's reality that success or failure in the lives of others greatly affects us. Someone's promotion makes us wonder why we haven't been promoted. Someone who suffers a great loss makes us better appreciate what we have, or possibly makes us dwell on a similar loss we've had. We are very good at comparing our life achievements and failures with those of others.

Thus, when you see someone pregnant, it is very hard not to compare their success to your own failure. It is an aggravating situation. If you are already on the verge of tears or anger, having someone solicit you for a baby gift might be enough to push you over the edge. You may try to hold back until the person soliciting you leaves before you break down. More likely, at least some of those emotions might be released as you say in clipped tones, "I don't have any dollar bills right now ..."

So, what can you do?

As with most things, there aren't any easy answers.

1. You can try to participate. As I said earlier, some people have that ability, and succeed at being magnanimous.

2. You can place a thick shell around yourself, such that things only bother you when you are alone and can let out a primal scream.

3. You can try to deal with each event as it arises, and hope that the people around you will understand what you are going through.

Dealing with Your Emotions

Choosing the third option, which is probably the most common one, is not an easy one to maintain. Depending on what you are going through, you might find it extremely hard to maintain your composure.

You'll have to determine, as with all things, who you can trust to see your emotions and whom you have to be circumspect with. If your boss doesn't understand your situation (even if you've told him or her), then you'll just have to be very careful in how you react around your boss. You might try to reserve showing your feelings until you are at lunch with someone you can trust.

Easy for us to say? Not really. Dealing with these issues is not easy. You won't always succeed. There will be days when you call in sick simply because you cannot face the world that day (and maybe there's a baby shower going on at the end of the workday). There will be days when you want to scream at the next person who interrupts you. There will be days when you just can't function.

That's true for many of the things mentioned earlier — deaths, sicknesses, and major events. But, until infertility is recognized more clearly by our society as a long-term event, you'll just have to deal with the fact that people will cut you much less slack than if you are dealing with a "socially recognized" event.

✧ ✧ ✧

The workplace has improved over time in recognizing that there are life events where you cannot be at work. Dealing with sick children during work became more acceptable only after enough women entered the workplace, meaning both parents were working when children became ill.

Your work environment determines which events are "socially recognized" as excusable absences. Depending on where you work, they can include sickness, vacations, sick children, deaths in the family, or maybe even golf on a sunny afternoon.

But, needing to go to the doctor to get artificially inseminated doesn't tend to go over as well. At best, it fits under the sickness category — at least you have to go see a doctor. But, you will often try your business compatriots' displeasure if you have to do it too often. Which you probably will have to do.

Most people will try to be patient. But after the tenth meeting missed, or the fifth time you have to ask someone to repeat themselves because the infertility medication is making you unable to concentrate; well, people tend to have a limited amount of patience.

They will slowly start moving their dependence from you to others. Yes, that will affect others opinions of your performance. And, it's not totally inappropriate; you probably aren't performing at the same level as before infertility started consuming your life.

It's also not totally fair because other "work affecting events" tend to be forgiven, at least to some degree. Hopefully, you are in an environment where the effects of your infertility on your performance are understood and accepted. But many of us are not that lucky.

✧ ✧ ✧

In the end, what can you do? The blithe answer is simply "the best you can," but that is probably also the only appropriate answer. In the end, you can only control yourself, not others. So, it continues to be your own responsibility to continue working if necessary, and to do the best job you can under these circumstances.

You probably should tell your manager of your situation. That way, absences, time away, and medication issues at least have an explanation. If you get an understanding response, be glad you have that manager. If not, you may need to tolerate what exists, look for a transfer, or even get another job.

Regardless of whether your manager understands or not, you need to take care of yourself. Don't neglect your sleep. If you have a deadline coming up, pushing yourself to extremes combined with the stress you are going through due to the infertility issue will only make you less efficient, not more. Similarly, you need to back off. Put your life, your work, and your activities into perspective. Focus on what is important. If you really need to get a deadline done, cut back on your activities, but not your sleep.

You are potentially going to get very little sympathy. Some people consider you less of a person if you admit to this problem. The sin of infertility strikes at times and your work prowess is questioned if you aren't fertile. If you have to deal with this, remember that this issue strikes even worse in other situations. There are much stronger prejudices than infertility.

If you are a man, you probably get even less sympathy, especially if you are the one going through medical treatment. Fertility is supposed to be a woman's problem. Many men will only denigrate you if you admit that this is an issue. After all, the comment "shooting blanks" is extremely derogatory. Once again, you'll have to carefully evaluate whom to tell. Who would be sympathetic to your issues about infertility?

At best, you will either have understanding co-workers and managers, or at least fellow employees who will learn to appreciate your situation. At worst, you will have people who are intolerant of your situation. In the latter case, these types of people are likely to be intolerant in situations other than infertility, and you will have to make the standard decision of "Am I better off working here, or not working here." Never an easy decision.

There is hope that changes in attitudes will continue to occur in the work environment about the needs of employees. If the needs of infertile couples become more broadly recognized, there will be more tolerance for them.

Overall, you spend over 25 percent of your time at work. It is a significant part of your life. You *will* have to deal with work during your infertility struggle. It won't be easy, but successfully keeping work from interfering with your struggle will go a long way toward helping you cope.

Notes

— Dealing with Work —

Dear Diary

Dan and Jan asked me to share my experiences at work with them. I thought the best way to do this would be to give them some of the entries in my diary. They are excerpts, of course, but should provide insight into what I've gone through by working during my infertility.

March 14

Today was my last day at work before getting married. Being at a small company is nice, because you know everyone, and they can throw the nicest bridal parties! I got some wonderful gifts, and they'll really help us as we get started in our marriage. I'm quitting, because we want to start a family right away, and I'm a strong believer in staying home with children. I don't want us to get caught in the trap of needing two incomes, so we're going to get by on Jim's alone.

March 22

My wedding day! It was a wonderful day. I know that a lot of people like to keep kids out of weddings, but I love kids! I'll have to admit that seeing the two little ring bearers come down the aisle with our rings was the absolute cutest — especially since they were Jim's baby brother and my baby sister. They looked like miniature versions of us.

Jim was so handsome in his tuxedo, and I think I looked pretty good in my gown as well. All in all, it went magnificently. A lot of my friends from work showed up, too, so it ended up being a pretty big wedding.

September 10

I never worried about my periods being variable before, but in the last few months, that fact has hit home with me. For a while, it didn't concern me, but I'm still not pregnant, and Jim and I decided I should see a doctor about it. The problem is that the doctor said I should start taking some drug to get my periods to be regular, and that I should keep seeing him for a while. But it is expensive, and Jim doesn't have any insurance that covers me going to this doctor.

October 5

Jim and I had a long talk today. We both agree I should keep seeing the doctor, but we figured out that the bills just are too high, and that the only way we can afford to do this is if I go back to work, at least until we get this all figured out. I guess that's fine with me, since my old company is willing to hire me back, even if it is in customer support instead of accounting. After I talked to them, they were willing to even have me come back starting tomorrow.

November 3

I never realized how hard it is to work when your mind is on something else. The drugs seem to have stabilized my periods, but now the doctor wants to do artificial insemination. The problem with that is I have to be in the doctor's office twice most of the morning next week. I've already used up all of my sick time; I started back out at zero when I restarted work, and I've had a couple of days where I stayed home because the drugs made me queasy. And I don't have any vacation accrued, either. I used what little I had of that, as well.

I went to my new boss about it; I offered to work extra hours in the afternoon to make up for the hours I'd have to miss. He was real huffy about it, saying things like "Customer support hours are 9 A.M. to 5 P.M. and that's when we need to be here," but he reluctantly said I could do some late afternoon work — maybe by helping the accounting department get caught up.

December 13

The Christmas party drove me crazy today! I've been avoiding the baby showers recently; it has just become too hard to go to them. It seems like *everyone* here is getting pregnant but me. What's even harder is being asked to donate to each baby shower when all of my salary is going to trying to *have* a baby.

But, I thought the Christmas party would be safe to go to. **Wrong!** Everyone was talking about presents for their kids, whether or not they should keep the kids believing in Santa Claus, new clothes for the new baby, etc. etc. etc. Now, maybe it really was just me, and that *wasn't* all they were talking about, but it sure seemed that way to me.

After a while, I started to just let all of that talk run pass me, but then one of my friends in Accounting walked in with her new baby. That happens once in a while given we are a small operation. I've usually been able to avoid it, since it tends to occur at baby showers and the like. But I couldn't avoid it now. I oohed and aahed along with everyone else, but I felt a stabbing in my stomach that wouldn't go away. I excused myself quickly thereafter, and went home as soon as I could.

January 14

My boss called me into his office today and blasted me for missing work. It seems like the extra work I was doing in accounting didn't really count, because I was "not available" during regular customer service hours too often. I tried to explain that it was a medical thing — I wasn't playing hooky or anything, I was in the doctor's office when I was missing work.

That didn't sit well with him. He was aware it was infertility treatments even though I hadn't really talked much about it. This was all "elective" and "my choice" and had nothing to do with really being sick. Thus, I was taking advantage of my position by being gone too often — my choice, it wasn't a medical thing, at least not to him.

I tried to explain that I was doing the best I could. Insurance didn't cover the treatments, I had to pay for all this myself, and I was trying to keep it from interfering with work. He just jumped on the fact that insurance didn't cover the treatments — which proved it was an elective thing, and had nothing to do with being sick, or being justifiably away from work.

I promised to talk to my doctor to see if we could keep my visits outside of work hours. The fact that my cycle might not allow that didn't seem to register with him; but my promise appeared to mollify him for the time being.

January 15

Well, I really stuck my foot in it this time. Another baby shower event comes my way, and I really said a mouthful. When asked to donate, I said "it's now my policy not to donate to non-work events; they don't contribute to the company." When asked "what did I mean by that," I said that if I couldn't take time to have a baby, why should other people be able to spend the last part of the day partying about having one? That certainly didn't go over well, and I regretted saying it right away. I wanted to explain further, to make it clear that I was really just hurting, but I got left alone pretty quickly after my statements.

February 23

Is the whole world pregnant? There are five women pregnant that are in the office. These days, it seems like women work until they deliver, and it is very obvious they are pregnant. A memo got put into everyone's cubicle — it went something like this:

"Don't Drink the Water Baby Pool" — "Greetings! Obviously, all you have to do around here to have a baby is to drink the water, so don't drink it if you don't want to get pregnant. Kristin, Hannah, Michelle, Laura, and Ashley are all going to have their babies sometime between March 1 and May 1. We're taking bets as to when each one delivers, and the one who gets closest overall will win the pot! The expected delivery dates are listed below, but we know you can come closer! Send your expected dates (don't forget hours!) to Bobbie via e-mail along with your $5 pool amount. Let's have fun with this!"

# Dealing with Your Emotions 193

Scribbled on my note were the words, "This is a non-work event, so don't bother ..." I was furious! Bobbie was the one who had come into my office in January, since she is the one who always seems to arrange these events. I had tried to apologize for my comments to her, but she had been extremely cool to me since then. I know she had also gossiped about my problems to others, and that she'd even discussed how our boss didn't think much about me, and how much I was missing work.

Now maybe I'm just being catty, but Bobbie doesn't work much on anything but these social activities. Of course, she's popular at work, since she helps the workplace be "fun." But I don't see how what she does is "ok," whereas what I need to do isn't.

February 25

E-mail was sent to everyone in customer service today from my boss. It said:

"There seems to be a lot of discussion and activity associated with the "Don't Drink the Water Baby Pool." Although I don't want to discourage camaraderie and having fun while at work, let me state that it is not appropriate to be betting within the office environment. Just as we don't sanction the basketball pools that have occasionally come up during office hours, we similarly cannot sanction any other events which involve gambling."

Everyone immediately blamed *me* for the E-mail. I hadn't done *anything*! But everyone just assumed that I must have complained about the pool, otherwise why would this message have come out? I didn't know what to say, and anyway, no one came directly to me to ask about it. I only learned about this from one of my close friends in accounting who passed on what the others in customer service were saying about me.

The only good thing about today was that my doctor said that he wanted to stop the artificial insemination for a while and instead to do some tests. The tests would be in the evening, so they wouldn't interfere with work. I had just about reached the end of acceptability for missing work certain mornings, so this was a welcome statement.

March 20

My boss came into my cubicle this morning and asked me to come into his office. He asked me if I had told my doctor that my boss didn't like me missing work. I said, "Well, yes, of course, that was how I could get him to try to rearrange my schedule." He said, "Did you know that your doctor and I are good friends? He called me today and said that I should excuse you from work and that it was necessary. Now, I respect the doctor-patient relationship, so I didn't ask why, but I wanted to let you know that if you need to miss work, it's ok."

I didn't know whether to feel good or bad about that — small towns are like that, I guess. But sure enough, when I got back to my desk, there was a voice mail from my doctor asking me to come into the office, today if possible.

When I got in, he told me that the tests had shown that I had cancerous polyps or something like that, and I would need to have them removed. I asked him what did that entail, and he said it probably meant a hysterectomy. I'd never be able to have children! I was only 28. Women my age didn't have hysterectomies! He scheduled the surgery for early next week.

March 22

Happy Anniversary! Jim surprised me with roses, and took me out to the fanciest restaurant in town. He gave me the prettiest card, and told me that I was the most important person in the world. I broke down crying right in the middle of dinner. He took me home, but he couldn't get me to stop crying. I'm crying right now while I write this. And I can't write anymore.

March 26

The surgery went well yesterday. I'm in a hospital bed, but they say everything went so well, I should be home by the weekend. My boss came to visit me this morning and asked how I was. I told him fine, but how could he justify visiting me during work hours? He smiled and said "Touché." Then he told me that he was taking a half-day of vacation so that it would be ok. He got quiet after that; he looked a lot older than he normally looked and he looked tired as well.

He said that Jim had told him what was going on, and that I would never be able to have my own children. He said some nice words about adoption, but when he said he understood, I couldn't help but snap, "You didn't understand when I needed to miss work!"

He said, "I'll forgive that outburst because I know what you are feeling. But I do understand. My only child Rob was killed in the Gulf War. I know what it means not to have any children. I had my only son taken away from me." He got up to leave, but turned and said, "And yes, I took a day of vacation to go to his funeral."

I think I liked it better when my boss was simply an ogre rather than a human being I just happen to disagree with.

April 10

Things haven't gotten much better at work. Everyone is trying to ignore what happened to me, especially since the contention between me and my co-workers dealt with babies and baby showers. The tiptoeing is as bad as or worse than the chilled atmosphere that was there before.

My boss seems to regret having shared his personal life with me. He only moved into town a few years ago, so I guess no one really knew about his son. I haven't told anyone but Jim about it, but my boss still isn't saying much to me.

Even though I am not going to the doctor for infertility treatments, there is still the follow-up to my operation. At least insurance covers that. Now I have to start thinking about adoption.

May 3

People have short memories, or maybe they just don't listen. The "Don't Drink the Water" baby pool, of course, just went underground after that e-mail. Turns out that Jeff Turner in accounting won the pool. Since I know Jeff, he was discussing winning the pool with me. "I was only off by a total of 180 hours for all five! Not bad, huh? So, are you drinking the water so I can bet on you, too?"

I just smiled. He walked away, totally oblivious to what he had said to me. I know he had heard about my operation, but either he had forgotten about it, or just didn't think about it.

Of course, I have to deal with it every day. I still can't go to baby showers. Maybe that will change once we adopt a child. I sure hope so.

— Accepting Others' Parenting Decisions —

You Can Do Better

Newspaper headlines can be difficult to read when they deal with the abuse of children. Babies in dumpsters, starving children in impoverished nations, children beaten or killed by their parents, or babies left in a car all day with the windows up.

"I could do so much better ..." you think. I would cherish and take care of my children better than the people portrayed by these events.

And, of course, you could. It's sometimes hard to remember that the events portrayed in such headlines are the extremes. You don't read about the majority of parents who are doing a good job in raising their children. Instead you read about the crashes and accidents of childhood tragedy.

But that doesn't change the fact that you wonder why people who abuse and misuse their children are "allowed" to have children. It seems unfair that some people can have children that they abuse when you can't have children that you would cherish.

The truth is that you cannot control how most children are raised. You are not responsible for the actions of others. What you can do better, though, is to address the individual instances around you. If an opportunity arises for you to make a difference in the life of a child, you need to decide if you have the time, ability, and desire to do so. This can include mentoring a child, contacting an agency in a case of child abuse, or becoming a foster parent.

This doesn't mean you should do more for children just because you happen to be infertile. These recommendations apply whether you are single, married with children, or a couple. When opportunity arises to improve your own or others' lives, you need to decide whether or not you can and want to be involved. Your infertility may make you more sensitive to the plight of abused or neglected children and therefore affect your decision to get involved or not, but infertility does not obligate you to do anything differently than you would if you were not infertile.

Your responsibility is to live your life in as positive a manner as you possibly can. If that involves improving the lot of children because you are sensitive to their issues, then that is good. If it does not, then direct your energies where they will be useful. It is perfectly appropriate to lament the improper decisions of others in how they raise their children, but it is not appropriate to dwell on it to the detriment of your own life.

You can do better by making the best choices you possibly can about your own life. If you have the energy and make the time, you can have an impact on how others make their decisions. Knowing this can help you understand the way of a world that includes the abuse of children. Understanding is not acceptance.

— Accepting Others' Parenting Decisions —

A Nightlight for Her Worries

Sarah's warm embrace and sweet, sweet smile
Belie her black eye and dirty clothes.
Another accident, of course.

She takes her seat and opens her books.
Expressive brown eyes you can drown in look at me.
Only seven, I marvel at her intelligence and attention.

I try to teach, but my eye continually finds her.
Her legs are still bruised, I can tell.
She can't quite hide the wounds with her dress.

Everyone knows the situation.
She basically raises herself,
though she lives with her mother and another man.

Authorities think they beat her,
But not enough is known.
I can only teach the little girl.

I try to make sure she eats a good lunch
since she is small and always hungry.
I can do little more.

I come home to my empty house.
My husband is away with his work.
I wish Sarah were here.

I would give her a nice meal, a warm bath,
A lap and some stories.
Hugs and kisses, tuck into bed,
A nightlight for her worries.

I don't pretend there would be no scoldings or time-outs.
Better those than screaming, beatings, and injuries.
I go to bed in the stillness, and pray once again for Sarah.
"Why isn't she mine, oh Lord?"
"Why don't they know the priceless gift you have given?"

I sleep, but not well.
School again, and all the precious children arrive.
But, today, Sarah is not here.

I silently pray that she is ok as I begin to teach.

— Giving Love to Pets —

Pets as Therapy

Pets can help you heal!

It is a general statement, but one most people agree is true. Pets can accept our love and give us unconditional love in return, thereby helping healing to occur.

A couple experiencing infertility is struggling with a lot of societal and personal issues, one of the strongest being feeling left out and alone.

While pets are not human, they can still become part of your family. In this fashion they can become surrogates for the children you desire. Pets can also be love surrogates to older people in nursing homes, or to a grieving person who has recently lost a spouse. Pets can help parents with empty nest syndrome, a child who wants a playmate, or someone whose love is far away.

In no way do pets replace the lost or missing object of our love and affection. They provide a place to cast your love — they receive your love and give love in return — they prevent us from withdrawing within ourselves, because they need our love and care.

As we meet their daily requirements, they make us feel needed. Pets never talk back to you or stop listening to you. Pets also know when you are hurting. They help you deal with your pain. A cat in your lap has the ability to absorb your tears.

Without pets, we often bottle up and hide part of the love we would give to a child. It is a silly playful love that we often do not share with a spouse because we are "all grown up." With a child or a pet we can let our guard down and be silly. We can tease. We can let loose our inhibitions, because we will not lose a pet's love if we do silly things.

In dealing with the stress of infertility, we can become so focused on our goal of having a child we forget we are full of love and need to share it. Pets help us share this love. They need us and we sense that need.

When we fill their needs by giving them love, they are happy.

A dog smiles, a cat purrs, a bird chirps.

— Giving Love to Pets —

A Knight in Shining Armor

When Tony met me for dinner on Wednesday he saw a great big smile on my face. As he sat down he wasn't sure what was going on, but he seemed glad I was so happy. Over the appetizers I showed him the pictures I had developed that day. He started laughing at the one of Sir Percival, our dog.

Sir Percival and I were lying on the bedroom floor amidst all of the bedding, asleep. It had been a hard day for me, and I had found Sir Percival sleeping on the laundry. Rather than scold him, I lay down beside him and fell asleep as well. Tony had found us there with Sir Percival's head resting on my outstretched arm. Only Sir Percival awoke when Tony snapped the picture, so it had been a complete surprise to me when I picked up the photos.

As we ate our salads, I told Tony that the picture had brightened my day at work. Whenever someone brought out baby pictures, I always had to sit quietly. But today, I was able to share Sir Percival's pictures at lunch. It started a whole series of pet stories. The stories got funnier and funnier and everyone had a good laugh.

Laughter is a wonderful way to spend a lunch hour. It is so much better than watching others talk about what you do not have.

As our dinner orders came, Tony commented on how I had been smiling the entire evening. He couldn't remember the last time our dinner had been as happy and relaxed — it seemed that recently we had only talked about our infertility treatments. Each month, more and more stress seemed to enter our lives as the treatments had so far been unsuccessful. It appeared that Sir Percival's presence had broken that conversational rut.

Sir Percival is one of the few joys that keep me going. My morning walk with him is always a delight. Sometimes the walk is fast and sometimes it is slow, but he insists we do it every morning. I even made him a raincoat for those days when the weather tries to keep us indoors. The walks keep me sane during my treatments and help me to think life through. With Sir Percival at my side, I feel loved.

Our dinner conversation continued to focus on Sir Percival. Tony mentioned that the first family member to greet him when he comes home from work is Sir Percival — love and affection rolled into a waggling body. We also reminisced about how Tony trained Sir Percival to collect the morning newspaper. Now, if Tony does not get up at the crack of dawn to let Sir Percival retrieve the paper, he gently nudges Tony with his nose. You could not ask for a better alarm clock. No barking, just gently nudging until you wake up and do as Sir Percival expects you to.

We reflected on how blessed we felt having our precious dog. At a time when we wanted to curl up and crawl within our shells, Sir Percival encouraged us to continue living.

Sometimes he brings me a smile simply by bringing me his favorite bone. I feel he must be complimenting me on being doggie enough to want a good bone to chew on or bury. He forces us to maintain our order and discipline, insisting that we feed and groom him; in return, he gives us a lot of love. His love is unconditional. When he wants to play and gives you that soulful look, you can't help but forget your troubles and give him attention. We know we are both the center of his universe. In all of this treatment stress, he has been one of our few releases from it all.

As Tony and I lounged after dinner with our coffee and dessert, we continued to remember good times with Sir Percival. Like his naming day. What a grand time we had! Along with our friends, we are into medieval history, so we decided to knight Sir Percival during a party. He was named "Finder and Rescuer of Fellow Humans Interested in Preserving the Sanctity of Medieval Times," distinguished for his pure heart and his valor. In hindsight, it was like some of our friends who chose a special name with meaning for their new baby. Sometimes they'd even have a naming ceremony for their child. Maybe Sir Percival was our child surrogate until our own was born.

Tony also pointed out that Sir Percival would always defend me. I had been recovering from some infertility surgery and was soaking up the sun in the back yard, when a stray dog that I still think might have had rabies entered our yard. Sir Percival stood carefully beside me growling and barking until the dog decided to find another way to go.

Upon realizing how much Sir Percival meant to us, Tony proposed a toast. He suggested we add to Sir Percival's list of titles and named him "Rescuer of Stressed Damsels and Giver of Warm Fuzzies." I agreed fully as we clinked our glasses together.

Dinner tonight was a smashing success. No arguing, no questioning, no stress. We need to do this more often. Our marriage needs it. I am glad Sir Percival can help us even when he is not present. He truly is my Knight in Shining Armor.

Notes

Part 5
Moving on with Your Life

Coping Mechanisms

    Distract Yourself with Life   209
    Velveteen Realities   213

Naming an Unborn Child

    What's in a Name?   215
    Petals in the Wind   217

Adoption as an Option

    Two Roads Diverged in a Wood, and I —   221
    Child of My Heart   225

Childless or Childfree?

    One Way or the Other   231
    The Chains of Freedom   235

What We've Gained

    Our Lives are What We Make of Them   239
    Freedom from Chains   243

Quote and references on page 213-214 are from the book
The Velveteen Rabbit
written by Margery Williams
First Publication Date: 1922

Quote on page 240 is from the prayer
Serenity Prayer
attributed to Reinhold Niebuhr (1930s).
Also attributed to Friedrich Oetinger (18th century) and others ...

— Coping Mechanisms —

Distract Yourself with Life

How many lives do you have? Well, unless you are a cat, or believe in reincarnation, your answer is probably just one. How many years do you have within that life? Let's hope it is at least seventy-five to a hundred, but we are keenly aware that our lives can end at any time.

The time you spend battling infertility not only cuts into the quantity of your life; it also takes its toll on the quality. Your emotions become frayed, your schedules controlled, and your body manipulated — all in the attempt to achieve that important goal of giving birth.

So how do you cope?

You use the day-to-day business of life to get through each day. You make the most of what you have. In other words, you distract yourself with your life.

Easy to say? Certainly. We admit that we didn't take as much advantage of life during our years of dealing with infertility as we would have liked. A lot of time simply "passed us by" as we allowed infertility treatments to consume most of our thoughts.

You need to take time to see what you enjoy and incorporate those things into your life.

Although "coping mechanisms" is the term normally used to label activities that make your life easier to deal with, we prefer to call these activities "living time." So much of our life is taken up by what we need-to-do. Dealing with infertility is something we need-to-do in order to have a child. At the same time, you also need to pay the bills, mow the lawn, work each day, as well as eat and sleep.

Your quality of life is improved each time you turn a need-to-do into a pleasant experience, into "living time." Do you enjoy cooking? Suddenly, meal preparation can become a joy. Do you like getting outside? Mowing and landscaping can become a hobby instead of a chore. Is your job fulfilling? Your career can become affirming to your well-being.

Of course, there are the easy "living time" activities. Are you a sports fan? Do you enjoy traveling? Are exercise, hiking, or gardening activities that make you happy? What are your hobbies? Do you collect coins or movies or art? Do you sew or build things or paint? The more time you make for those things that simply give you pleasure, the better your quality of life.

We hear you saying "But there isn't enough time in the day! I have so many things that I need-to-do that I don't have time for the things I'd like to do. I know I need to relieve my stress, but I don't have enough time!" We understand and sympathize. We fall into the same rut of prioritizing the things we need-to-do ahead of the things we'd like to do. And this becomes especially acute when you add the need for infertility treatments to the mix.

As best as you can, you need to reprioritize. Ask yourself if you really have to deal with *all* the needs you've added to your list. If you are saying yes, stop reading this book, and go write down all the things you need-to-do during the next week. If you can't find something to cut back on, it's time to reanalyze what you are doing to yourself above and beyond infertility issues.

Remember that you only have one life to live. We guarantee you will not remember the deadline you made on Project #722 at work. You will not care that you mowed every week. Instead, you will remember things that gave your life meaning.

You will not remember the things you had to do. You will remember whether or not you enjoyed your life. And, yes, you will remember whether or not your infertility treatments were successful, because those do strongly affect the outcome of your life, but you cannot let that be the only thing you remember.

✧ ✧ ✧

Moving on with Your Life

As you begin adding "living time" to your life, don't let these items turn into another list of need-to-dos. Items that may initially add to your life can become obsessions rather than coping mechanisms. For example, you may join a club in order to have fun, but soon find yourself serving as president, putting out the newsletter, and being too busy to enjoy the activity. Once "living time" becomes a need-to-do, it is no longer a plus in your life.

In coping with infertility, make sure your "living time" includes discussing your trauma and pain with someone who can understand and who will listen. Letting your troubles out is a way of coping.

Finally, there is one way of coping with infertility that you may not have considered. Kids. If you can enjoy other people's children, you may find that goes a long way toward giving you patience as you work toward having your own. The key issue here is the same as with all "living time" activities — can you enjoy being with children as you deal with trying to have your own? If not, don't add it to your list.

Some women find babysitting other people's preschool children an effective method of coping with the fact that they haven't yet had children of their own. In our own case, neither of us could handle having babies around, but we received great enjoyment having our niece visit us for three weeks every summer from the time she was ten until she turned fifteen.

We've also been surrogate uncle and aunt to quite a few of our friends' children. Given our own consideration of "living time," once they passed five, some of these children would even stay overnight at our house. We'd play cards and games with them, and enjoy having children for a while. The bottom line was that children were in our lives during the period where we were trying to have our own.

There are many coping mechanisms available to you. Hobbies. Leisure activities. Vacations. Sports. Turning work into play. Turning chores into fun. Talking with others to release your feelings. Taking advantage of other people's children to enrich your life. All of these things are important ways to cope with your infertility. They are great ways to cope with any of your problems.

Choose whatever works the best for you, but be sure to add some "living time" to this stressful period of your life.

— Coping Mechanisms —

Velveteen Realities

Have you ever read *The Velveteen Rabbit*? This wonderful little book is about toys, memories, and wishes, but most of all, it's about being **real**.

A little toy Velveteen Rabbit is loved and treasured so much by a little boy that, as the "Skin Horse" says, "**Real** isn't how you are made. It's a thing that happens to you. When a child loves you for a long, long time, not just to play with, but *really* loves you, then you become *real*."

Right after we started our infertility treatments, Denise found a "deluxe special package" containing a copy of the book as well as an actual Velveteen Rabbit, probably about the same size as intended in the story. The box had a plastic cover wrapped with ribbon so you could see what was inside.

Instead of opening it, Denise said, "That's for our first child. I want our baby to have a Velveteen Rabbit, so that they can make it *real*." So the box went into the closet, and as the years went by, I more or less forgot about it.

Friends were still aware that we enjoyed the book, and during our infertility struggle I personally got a nice hardback copy from a close friend, signed "For the Kid in You." Even that was years ago, and strangely enough, I never read that copy of the book until tonight. Reading it is painful to me, because it reminds me that we don't have children to make velveteen rabbits *real*.

We've moved quite a few times over the last few years. Recently, I made a promise to myself to go through each and every last box and to throw away all of the junk we haven't used. As I was performing this task, a knot began to well up in my throat. Old memories. Items that had been put aside and forgotten. Denise's little velveteen rabbit came to mind, and I *knew* what would be contained in the very next box ..., a half-crushed package, covered by a cracked plastic cover.

Abandoned, without an owner, the rabbit would still be waiting.

Waiting to be used. Waiting to be loved. Waiting to be *real*.

✧ ✧ ✧

Strangely enough, I got to the last box, and never found it. Yet I knew it had not been discarded, but had survived every single move. When I mentioned it to Denise that night in bed, she got out of bed without saying a word, opened her clothes closet, and pointed way up top to a box, which loudly proclaimed on the side, "Love makes you *real*."

I climbed up on a stool and carefully took the box down. Rather than being crushed and bent, the box was in perfect condition, but still, never opened.

"Do you want to open it?" asked Denise.

"No," I answered. Carefully, I placed the unopened box back into the top of her closet.

There, the rabbit still waits.

"And while the Boy was asleep, dreaming of the seaside, the little Rabbit lay among the old picture-books in the corner behind the fowl-house, and he felt very lonely."

— Naming an Unborn Child —

What's in a Name?

In human society, a person becomes someone when he or she has a name.

Many couples buy books that list tens of thousands of names accompanied by a description of their meaning, the language they are derived from, and the multitude of individual spellings they might have. In addition, the most popular names are tabulated, cross-referenced, and published yearly.

Some parents give their children a name that fits into their prevailing culture and society so they won't be thought weird or abnormal. Others look for a name that is altogether different so that their child will be unique. Names are also used to observe family tradition. Passing on a name that has been used in a family for generations can cause "Jr." or "III" to be a mark of family pride. Middle names are often used to preserve a woman's maiden name through her child. Names that have become less popular over time, but that still mark a family's heritage; also tend to find a place in middle names.

We feel special when we hear our name called, or see it in print. By the same token we are offended when our name is misspelled or left out when we feel it should be included. We respond when someone calls our name, even if that person is calling someone else by the same name. The importance of our name is emphasized in studies showing that soldiers whose names were called more often during mail call were able to cope better with stress. They had a greater sense that someone cared for them in a special way.

In short, names are powerful.

For these reasons it is therefore totally appropriate to name an unborn child even if the child does not survive to live in our world. A child is a child, regardless of how long it lives. Without attempting to discuss or argue when life begins, it is sufficient to say that if one perceives that life existed, then a name for that life, however short, is an appropriate step to take.

When we find out we are pregnant and we want to be pregnant, happiness, excitement, and joy fill our bodies and minds. Once we perceive that we have a child, that child needs a name if we want the child to be more "real" to us, even if only in our memories.

Many people experiencing infertility are able to conceive a child, but then lose the baby before birth. Upon the loss of a baby, there is grieving, pain, and a strong feeling of loss. Giving that baby a name is one way to acknowledge that baby's existence by turning what was a pregnancy into a child, rather than keeping the pregnancy as an event.

For some it is more comfortable to maintain the pregnancy as an event by naming it "my miscarriage," "my second pregnancy," "my tubal pregnancy," or "my blighted ovum." Instead of a personal name, it can be a coping mechanism to label the pregnancy in medical terms rather than emotional ones.

In deciding whether your pregnancy was a child or an event, you may find comfort in leaving the issue alone for a while. Over time, as you cope, you will decide how to remember your loss.

It is normal and healthy to acknowledge and grieve for a lost child, born or unborn. By naming your unborn child, the child exists in your universe. And if you believe in an afterlife, you can envision them in heaven, pray for them, and hope to one day see them again. It is one way to acknowledge your loss, and to begin healing. If you consider your pregnancy to be a child, don't be afraid to choose a name to honor that remembrance. If you don't know the baby's sex, choose a neutral name. In our society, a person is known by their name. You need to decide whether naming that child will help you as you continue to live life.

— Naming an Unborn Child —

Petals in the Wind

The sun was beginning to rise as we approached the small park near our house. Hannah, finally fully awake, asked if she could swing on the swing set.

"No, honey, remember, it's Zachary's day," I said. Only three-years-old, she didn't fully understand, but she felt my serious mood and followed me to the small glade of wildflowers. The grass was damp with morning dew, but I sat down anyway, wanting to be closer to nature.

I placed the small box I had carefully carried with me in my lap. Hannah nestled up next to me, satisfied and quiet for the moment.

And I remembered.

✧ ✧ ✧

The pain had kept on and on. I guess they were contractions, but at four months into my long-awaited pregnancy, I didn't expect to have contractions. Tom kept hoping the pain would stop. After a while, we felt it was an emergency. Our doctor confirmed it when he told us he would meet us at the hospital immediately. We had tried for three years to get pregnant and although we were worried, we told ourselves this was normal and that if I lay quiet, the pains would stop.

After we arrived at the emergency room, everything seemed to happen in fast motion. Ultrasound showed the baby was not doing well. My cervix was dilating and I was in the middle of a miscarriage. I kept pleading with God to let our baby live, but I was filled with a deep sense of despair.

With my very encouraging husband, and capable and understanding doctor, I delivered our son. People asked me how I could call this fetus a child, a son. After all, he was only four months along. I couldn't tell them how I held our dead child on my chest and how we had a beautiful, perfectly formed little boy. Everything we saw was formed. Little hands, little feet, a mouth, eyes. He was just a smaller version of what he would have been later on had I been able to carry him five more months.

It was very strange, being in a hospital, holding our premature, dead child. A child we had so much hope for. When he was born, I was in a lot of pain and grief. I'll admit that I was less than grateful that the nurse not only insisted we hold the child, but also that we have pictures taken. But now I thank that nurse often in my thoughts.

A sort of numbness set in as they took my baby away. Our doctor wanted some testing done immediately to determine why the early birth happened. Hopefully, we could prevent it in any future pregnancies.

Before they took the baby, hospital officials asked us if we wanted to have a funeral. Did we want the baby cremated? It was hard enough focusing on what had just happened, much less making decisions for the future. By way of an answer, we told them to cremate the baby, adding that we did not know if we would have a funeral or not.

Finally, I fell into a deep sleep, while Tom slept in the chair next to me. The next day as Tom and I talked about our child through tears, we decided to bury him. It would allow us to acknowledge that we had given birth to a baby boy and would give us a tangible memory when we visited the gravesite.

Unfortunately, we learned that the baby had been cremated during the night. Knowing that I had said to do that, I asked if I could at least have the remains in an urn. The response was that with a child so young there were not enough minerals in the bones to leave remains. If I had told them, they could have wrapped the child in a baby blanket so there would be some residue. Admittedly the residue was from the blanket, but it was something. We started grieving afresh.

The next few weeks were difficult. The nursery, already set up with family antiques, seemed more than empty. After a few months, I started taking Clomid again; the doctor was optimistic since we had been able to get pregnant.

Time passed. In an antique store one day, I saw a small lacquered box decorated with dozens of tiny cherubs. For a moment, I imagined my little boy, up in heaven, among those cherubs. Then it struck me that it was one year ago that day that I had delivered my baby.

I'm sure the clerk wondered why my face was full of tears as I purchased that box. When I got home, I was surprised to find a dozen roses on the dining room table with a small card from Tom saying, "I didn't forget."

That evening, as Tom held me and promised me that I would be pregnant soon, I told him that I didn't even know our baby's name. He said that was ok, because God and we would always remember him. Later that evening, we named him Zachary.

After a few days, I carefully took each petal from the roses Tom had given me and placed them and some desiccant in the lacquered box. The cherubs on the lid appeared to be smiling as I did so.

Our lives went on. Over time, most everyone forgot how I had miscarried, especially once I became pregnant with Hannah. Zachary, by the necessity of life and time, became a footnote to our everyday living. But once a year, Tom gives me a dozen roses and I always put the petals in my special box. And once a year, now, I come to this park and remember.

✧ ✧ ✧

The wind has picked up as it has every year for the past six years. I awaken Hannah, who had fallen asleep at my side.

"Are you ready?" I ask.

I open my little box of cherubs and toss the rose petals high into the air. The wind picks them up and carries them along its currents. Hannah giggles and chases after them.

I silently tell the petals to find Zachary. Tell him I remember. My baby has gone where the dew goes when the sun shines. He's where the wind is on a calm day. I tell the petals that they can find him there.

And tell him I will never forget.

— Adoption as an Option —

Two Roads Diverged in a Wood, and I —

How long have you been trudging on the road of infertility? At some point, if you still have not had a biological child, you will begin to consider having a child a different way.

Most people don't think about adoption until they have to deal with it personally. Some people consider adoption whether they are fertile or infertile. However, most infertile couples only consider adoption after they discover they are unable to have a biological child. People's emotions vary greatly about this topic. Some want to adopt, some don't and some will if that is the only way they can parent. It is a touchy issue for some people; for others, it is an obvious solution to infertility.

Infertile people go through many emotions when they discuss adoption. It is important to acknowledge and examine these emotions and differences of opinion before adoption occurs as they can otherwise cause serious problems later on. As a couple, you need to decide why you want a child. In addition to giving and receiving love and affection, what are the other reasons you want a child? Is it to achieve genetic continuity? To nurture? To mentor? To teach? To have someone who depends on you?

In trying to reach a decision, couples find they first need to answer two questions:

"How much do we want to parent?"

"Are we more concerned with the pregnancy and birth experience or with the raising of a child, regardless of whether it is a child we have biologically conceived, birthed and are now going to nurture to adulthood?"

In discussing these issues, you should deal with intense questions like the meaning of life and parenting in general. Why do you even want to be parents? In considering adoption, you need to understand that you may be about to take an entirely new path on the road of life. Since we have not adopted and are not experts on adoption, we strongly encourage you to seek out books on this topic, just as we encouraged you to seek out books on the medical treatments available to get pregnant.

Adoption involves as many disparate issues as infertility. It is another way to have a child, but it is not simple. You have to consider open vs. closed adoptions, agency vs. private adoptions, being examined by social service groups, infant vs. toddler vs. older adoption, biracial and international adoption, etc., etc. Just as there are support groups for infertile couples, there are support groups for people considering and pursuing adoption. We encourage you to seek them out just as we encouraged you to investigate groups like RESOLVE.

Adoption brings up a whole new set of issues that you will need to deal with to achieve the child of your dreams, including the following:

How much red tape are you willing to go through to parent a child?

Are you going to continue infertility treatments as you pursue adoption? If so, realize that you will have to deal with the energy required to pursue infertility treatments as well as the energy to pursue adoption.

If you end up having a biological child as well as an adopted child, do you think there will be an issue in your household?

Are you ready to be checked out to see if you are fit to be a parent? Many adoptions involve showing that you can properly raise a child. This is not a bad thing, since the child's interests are paramount. Nevertheless, it causes many infertile couples to wonder why fertile couples don't have to qualify to be "fit" parents.

You also need to realize that there are issues about how people look at adopted children, apart from how you look at the role. Your parents may agree or disagree with your decision. Your friends may ask why you adopted the child you did. You will be second-guessed and asked

Moving on with Your Life

to explain no matter what you do. For example, if you ***only*** want a healthy infant, you may be perceived as selfish. Only a few will understand that being infertile doesn't suddenly add you to the small list of special people who choose to raise children not in the "healthy infant" category. For most people, the ability and patience required to handle a special needs child is an extraordinary one. When this role is thrust upon them through mental and physical disabilities, for example, everybody does the best they can, but it isn't a role sought out by most people. We applaud those who have the love to do this. Oddly enough, though, if you are infertile and even if you do not believe you have that necessary ability or patience, you may still be branded as "selfish" for only wanting a child without these attributes.

Remember that adoption is for children, not adults. The purpose is to provide a safe, stable environment for the child. Therefore while you may benefit by being able to parent a child that you may not have been able to parent without adoption, it is the child who should receive the major benefit.

Our society agrees with that concept, but is still trying to come to grips with "what is best" for children involved with adoption. There is a tendency to believe that the biological parent is always the best person to raise the child if he or she desires to do so. This is a correct assumption in most cases.

Unfortunately, there are publicized cases of children being taken from their adoptive homes. This is deterring some potential parents from adopting, since they believe they are perceived as "second best" compared to genetic parents. That widespread perception also needs to be considered as you pursue adoption.

As you can see, there are as many uncertainties and issues on the adoption path as there were on the infertility path. You will deal with some of these issues for the rest of your life.

Does that mean you shouldn't pursue adoption? Of course not! You have already expended the energy necessary to pursue having a biological child. If you still desire to parent, taking the adoption road might be exactly what you need to do in order to fulfill your long-desired goal of being a parent.

In the end, you need to choose the path that is right for yourself. You need to decide whether adoption is right for you. We strongly encourage you to consider this option if you have a strong desire to parent, but have been unable to have a biological child.

— Adoption as an Option —

Child of My Heart

My name is Susan Perkins Anderson. I'm thirty-two years old, born on August 17. I was married eleven years ago on June 4. My husband's name is Christopher Timothy Anderson. He's thirty-four and his birthday is May 15. Genealogy is my hobby. Can you tell?

I've been interested in my genealogy since I was a child. My great-grandmother Ada would tell me stories about her growing up, and about the Perkins family. Ada is my father's father's mother. I was always fascinated by her stories, and when I became a teenager I'd write down the stories, and get information on when everyone was born, married, and died. Gramma Ada has a terrific memory, and even now at ninety-five, she can still recall many dates and stories.

I have over fifteen hundred names in my computer genealogy program. I have all of my Dad's family, brothers, sisters, etc. I have my direct Perkins line back to 1655 when John Perkins came to Massachusetts from England. It gets interesting as you go further back; the dates get cloudy, information becomes unclear, and sometimes people end up missing, wrong, or out of place.

Folks used to have big families. I'm an only child, and maybe that, combined with the genealogy searching, made me want to have a big family of my own. Five children? Sure. More? Maybe so!

Chris also wanted a big family, so when we got married we immediately got started. Or we tried to get started. Yes, I'm infertile. I've been to doctors, done the medical stuff, Chris has been tested, we've done the charts, etc. Despite all this, nobody really knew why we couldn't have children.

Not having children has made me delve more into my genealogy, especially the Perkins genealogy. My Perkins family has a proud heritage — nothing spectacular, but the family is one you can be proud of. Even though I wouldn't have been passing on the name directly, all of my children's middle names would definitely have been Perkins.

After a while, our infertility became obvious, even though Chris and I didn't talk about it. I was staying home to have children. Everyone knew we wanted children. So rather than talk about the subject directly, relatives and folks started wondering if we planned to adopt. (That way, they were able to skip past all the infertility conversations.)

Chris seemed more amenable to adopting than I was. I wanted to give birth! I wanted to have *my* baby. And, yes, I wanted to pass on my heritage. I could imagine an adopted child. I'd love the baby, nurture it, raise it, and then when they were almost grown, my greatest fear was that they'd want to go find *their* parents, *their* heritage. All of my work and love would be cast off in favor of who they *really* were.

I don't think I'm being paranoid. Everyone reads about children who want to find out who their *real* parents were. I guess parents who adopt aren't *real* enough. So whenever anyone brought up adoption, I'd say, "No, we're going to have our own children some day."

I guess that's what kept me on the medications; that's what kept me going through all those trying times when my period would come, and I knew I still wasn't pregnant. I'm still fairly young, so I keep hoping, but the doctors seem to have given up on me, except those who are willing to do anything as long as we keep paying them. The more honest ones say things like "progesterone level problems" and "egg follicle something or other" and tell me that maybe I should adopt.

Gramma Ada didn't totally understand what I was going through. She has a terrific memory, but she gets a little confused about what is going on in the present. And the fact I wouldn't discuss what was on my mind didn't help. But she knew I had been upset during our last few visits together, and she knew how much I liked genealogy and family stories, so she had a major surprise for me during our last visit.

"I never wanted to give this to you before, because I wanted to make sure I gave it to someone who would take care of it as much as I have.

Your father, grandfather, and your aunts never really cared, but I think you do," she said mysteriously as she kept drumming her fingers on a large cardboard box.

I almost screamed when she opened it. I never knew there was a "Perkins Family Bible"! And letters! Scads of letters from long ago. It was an absolute treasure trove.

"Why didn't you give this to me before? It would have made my research so much easier." I couldn't help but ask.

"Why, then, you might not have been as willing to listen to an old lady tell her old stories," answered Gramma Ada. "You'll see that some of my stories come from these letters. And didn't you wonder how I always knew the correct dates? I'm not a dumb old lady, and I like your company. Giving you this might have made you less willing to come over, listen, and tape record my voice. Tut, tut! Don't try to deny it. But I've always loved you, and I don't know how much longer I'll be around, so I wanted to make sure you had this. You've seemed upset lately, so I wanted to give you something I thought you'd like."

Thought I'd like? Wow. As I was leaving, I reassured her that having this material wouldn't keep me from visiting, and I rushed home. The next few nights involved reading letters, scanning the birth and death dates in the Bible, and just absorbing all of it. Gramma Ada was right in one sense. I didn't get much new information as she had given me most of it in her stories, but it was exhilarating just holding this in my own hands.

The seventh night after Gramma Ada had given me the Bible and letters, I started my period. This cycle hadn't worked either. Chris started talking about discontinuing the treatments. He was concerned about how they were affecting me. I wasn't the happy person he'd married, he said. Of course, not! How could I be happy when we couldn't have children?

He told me he'd been doing research on adoption and said that he thought it would be a good idea. He even pulled out a couple of pro-adoption books that he thought I might like.

Having just started my period, I blew up! I told him that we were going to have *our* children, and that was that. That next time it would work and that I'd have a baby and it would be *our* baby. I didn't want to have to raise someone *else's* baby.

Then I ran into the guest bedroom where I had carefully laid out all the letters and my notes. I grabbed the Bible and opened it to the birth and death dates. I started tracing my finger over the birth dates of those who had come before me. I saw my own name that Gramma Ada had put in the Bible thirty-two years before. It stunned me when I realized that I was the *last* generation on the chart. Since this was a five-generation set of descendants, there was no room for anyone else. That had never bothered me before, but given what had happened, I started crying.

Chris came in and took the Bible away. "You wouldn't want to get tears on this," he said gently. He'd never really looked at the Bible before, since he knew how carefully I took care of it. Now, he glanced at why I had been crying, and started paging through the large book. He didn't say anything as I regained my composure, but as he handed the Bible back to me, he idly said, "What's in the back cover?"

"What?" I quipped, not sure what he meant.

"The back cover. There's stuff inside."

I'm not sure why I'd never noticed it before, but the back cover *was* thick. I guess I'd assumed it was padding. But the front cover wasn't like that, and upon further investigation we found that the back cover had been carefully stitched together. There were more papers inside. Chris guessed that Gramma Ada had probably put them there, but when I asked her later, she said that she didn't know about them. My best guess is that the papers had been carefully put in there by my great-great grandmother, Gramma Ada's husband's mother, who had the Bible before Gramma Ada.

I immediately imagined some deep dark secret being revealed. It felt like a murder mystery or something. "The secret papers found in the family Bible." Imagine my shock when my thoughts were indeed verified; the papers were adoption papers! It turns out that my great-grandfather, William Perkins, was *adopted* by my great-great-grandparents. William was Gramma Ada's husband. I wasn't a Perkins after all! This was definitely a deep dark secret, because I know that no one knew about this, at least not in the present day.

Suddenly I had the awful feeling that all my research was going to have to start over again. That my genealogy back to 1655 was a sham. That I had to really dig down and find out who William's parents really were, because that information had been carefully eradicated from the adoption papers. This revelation both depressed and energized me. I wanted to know more, so I re-read my great-great-grandmother's diary (which was one of the "letters" in the box) very carefully for signs about the adoption, and maybe to find out her thoughts about it. She never mentioned it specifically, but I found one passage that I think is very telling:

> *I love all my children dearly.*
> *All four of them are extremely special to me.*
> *But I will always feel that my second oldest, William,*
> *holds a special place in my thoughts.*
> *I guess you could call him the 'Child of My Heart'*
> *since he captured my heart from the time he was born.*

I carefully held the old diary as I tried to envision my great-great-grandmother writing this passage. I had only seen her picture in old photographs. She had hidden an adoption in the back of a family Bible. Why? Here I was performing William's role of wondering who I *really* was.

Was she concerned that her son might search for his real parents? Did she think he might consider himself less a part of the Perkins family had he known? Did she consider her hiding of the evidence as a sin or a blessing? I sat for quite a while, reading the passage over and over, not knowing who I was or what I belonged to.

Suddenly, it didn't seem to matter. I was still a Perkins. My family had been raised as Perkins, all the way back to 1655 and earlier. Adoption didn't change that. I was still me. My great-great-grandmother was who she was. And William was and always would be one of her four children, whom she loved.

I walked into the living room where Chris was watching a ball game. He started to protest when I grabbed the remote and turned the TV off, but he quieted when I put my finger on his lips.

"Could you let me see those adoption books you read?" I asked. "I'm still not sure, and I still want to keep trying, but I think I want to have a 'Child of My Heart'."

— Childless or Childfree? —

One Way or the Other

Are you still with us? Still traveling that infertility road, wondering when you'll finally have children? There does come a time when you have to ask yourself if it is time to stop the medical treatments you've been undergoing to have children. You've worked hard, but you haven't achieved your goal. Maybe you never managed to get pregnant or you lost your child. You cannot get to a resolution in this matter.

Maybe it is time to change the rules.

When you started down the infertility road, you described your situation something like "We are having a few problems in having children, but we're going to work it out soon." Over time, it shifted to "We don't have any children, but we are still working on it." Now, as you continue to get older, your efforts yield only a description of "Childless, but still trying to change the situation."

You may be tired of actively trying to change the situation. Does that mean you are left being childless? Only if you choose so! You could move onto the path of adoption, but if adoption is not right for you, you can still change the rules. You can decide to be *childfree* as opposed to *childless*.

Semantics, you say? It's all semantics? Is there really a difference between *childless* and *childfree*? Both terms mean that you don't have the child you have tried so long to have.

So who cares what you call yourselves? *You* should care. Certainly, the difference between childless and childfree is within your state of mind. Both mean that you do not have any children. In both cases, there will be an ache in your heart for what might have been. There will be times when you dream of how you could have cuddled your child in your lap, soothed a hurt, or taught something new and wonderful to a small trusting soul for whom you were responsible.

But if you can embrace the idea of changing the rules, you can accept the title *childfree* rather than *childless*. There are other roads to travel. There are other directions for you to take that are as rewarding and fulfilling as raising and mentoring a child. You may have become so focused on having a child that this concept is foreign to you. "Is there really something else I can do?" you ask. Amazingly, there are many important things in life that have nothing to do with children. And you can choose to pursue one or several of these paths.

"But, but, what about children? Do I have to abandon that dream?" If you want to be childfree rather than childless, yes, in a sense, you do abandon that dream.

In order to call yourself childfree, you can no longer dwell on having children. If you have baby furniture, you put it away, give it away, or sell it. You make a decision to stop medical treatments. You may even go on birth control to enforce this decision upon yourself. (No, we can't imagine that either, but we're trying to cover all bases.)

The point is that you are moving away from the efforts required to have children and developing new areas within your life. The more you look back, the more your mindset is in the childless arena. The more you look to other areas within your life, the more you are in the childfree mindset.

This does not mean that you no longer want children. You can continue to have sex. If you have "unknown" infertility, a low sperm count, or irregular periods, you may continue to entertain an occasional hope or dream of a child you may have some day. But you need to view this hope or dream similar to winning the lottery. That is, to be childfree, a pregnancy would come as a surprise, not as the result of your efforts. Otherwise, your mindset has not moved to new areas in which to enrich your life. If you have tried to live childfree but find yourself continuing to dwell on children, don't forget that you can change your mind and go back to trying to have a child.

Ambivalence is ok for a while. In fact, it is a necessary step as you gradually move from "really trying" to have children to the "not trying" to have children lifestyle. This ambivalence may be fine, even for a few years. But don't forget that your life is somewhat on hold as you move back and forth trying to make a final decision. You should not live only for the hope of having children. At some point, you have to make a choice.

Making that choice can be empowering. After all, you have been denied the choice to have children. Maybe it is time you took charge of your life again. You *can* choose your path in life, rather than having your choices forced upon you. Finally, *you* can decide.

Notes

— Childless or Childfree? —

The Chains of Freedom

Looking back, all those treatments seem like a nightmare. They never worked, and we never became pregnant. It was a relief when we finally decided to be childfree. Our therapist tried to get Bobby and me to discuss the five stages of grief, but I already knew we were in the last stage: Acceptance.

I knew that we were not going to have children, and that it was time to get on with our lives. We needed some event to separate our infertile time of life to our new life of childfree living, so we decided to take that trip to Europe we had been delaying for so long because of infertility treatments.

I remember thinking this would be a wonderful transition. We were finally going to stop treatment! We were going to Europe to celebrate the event. We had finally made a decision! All the treatments had been for nothing and adoption didn't seem right for us. We were so sure that we would conceive our own biological child that taking someone else's baby did not feel right.

As part of our planning, our therapist suggested we clean out the baby's room before we went, but that didn't make sense. Besides, it would not be right if we finally conceived after all. We would just close the door for now.

I remember the day we had gone to that quiet place in the mountains before we reached our final decision. It seemed that no matter where we went, we talked about getting pregnant. We were obsessed. Even when we snuggled we wondered if this would be the time we would conceive. Now, just four months later, we decided we were going to stop treatments forever. We were never going to have children! It was the best decision, really. The treatments were tearing us apart. We seemed to argue so much compared to when we weren't trying. And if we could recapture the innocent days and our happiness with each other, it would be wonderful. Maybe this trip to Europe would help us to do that. Now we could end our obsession.

As I packed for Europe, many thoughts raced through my mind. What clothes would we need? How many evening gowns should I take? What kind of restaurants would we eat at? How about those after-theater parties? Would we really be able to get around without knowing the language? Thank goodness we had a good travel agent who answered all our questions.

While I packed the electrical converters and essential toiletries, I wondered again if we had made the right decision to stop infertility treatments. I thought back to the grieving process that our counselor had tried to make me memorize. Sometimes it hurt so much that I did not want to deal with it. I was glad we were going to get past all that after this trip. No treatments meant that we could happily live childfree. Besides, we just might be able to conceive on our own if we weren't under all of this pressure to perform each month. And who knows, maybe after we had relaxed for a while, we would have the energy to do one more treatment. After all, our insurance does cover 90 percent. Anyway, for now we were on our way to something new and exciting.

As we walked through the airport, I noticed this huge panda bear at the cutest little shop. It was sort of like the panda I grew up with and told my troubles to. We just had to have it for the nursery! I convinced Bobby to buy it. It was so cute that I could not think of stuffing it into a box to send home, so I told the sales clerk that I would carry it. It was so smooth and cuddly and comforting. When we had our baby, I knew she would like her just as much as I did right now.

When we stepped off the plane, everything was so different. The clothes! The people! The smells! The sights! It was so exciting and new! We were ushered into customs with me carrying our baby's panda, and I remember as we went out seeing a group of people with infants crying. I wondered if this is what my friend Cheryl was talking about when she mentioned foreign country adoptions. What a trying way to get a child.

Seeing Frankfurt was a joy. The buildings were so old, and everyone seemed to move a little slower than back home in the states. As we took the train into the countryside I marveled at how clean everything was. There were no billboards on the roadsides, and each farm looked so picturesque.

When we got off of the train, at our first stop we started looking for our bed and breakfast. The landlady admired our panda. She said it would grace our bed most beautifully. After we got settled in, we went in search of breakfast and that is when I lost my composure. Seeing lots of women with their children in the town square going to market, I realized I had no family and never would. I started sobbing and Bobby tried to quiet me, saying that I was making a scene and I should control myself. What did I have to cry about? We were here in Europe enjoying ourselves!

When we got back to the hotel and found the panda proudly sitting on our bed, I felt like a fool. I was just kidding myself when we bought that panda. We'd never have children! Where were the children we should have had? Why did the peasant women in town deserve five children each when we had none? Bobby just stood watching me cry into the panda. I wish he understood my pain.

I wondered if the pain would ever go away. Would I ever get used to being without children? How do other couples become childfree? Everyone at work thought we were so lucky to be able to take such a nice vacation.

Thinking back on that trip, most of it was a blur. I remember that I did put on a happy face for Bobby as we saw the sights. I felt like everyone was staring at a woman who wasn't really a woman. I couldn't be worth anything if I couldn't bear my husband an heir! I had thought getting away and doing something new would be healing. Was I wrong! We should have done something more healing, like going to the beach and just lying in the sun.

When we returned home one of the first things we did was put the panda in its room, our baby's nursery. Seeing the panda in its rightful place felt more healing than the entire European trip. Some day our child would be thrilled to hold her panda. I'm glad we did not take the therapist's advice and clean out the room.

Back at work, all my co-workers are excited to see our pictures. They seem so envious and say that they wish they had gone before their children came. Now, they would be lucky to go after the children got through college. I just smile because we were lucky enough to go now. Maybe delaying having children will enable us to be better parents when our child is born. Maybe it is good that we are currently childfree and that we accept that fact without any problems.

— What We've Gained —

Our Lives Are What We Make of Them

Here we are at a crossroads in the journey of life. We're all here, it seems. We see those who dealt with infertility for a while but finally had a child. We see newly adoptive parents. We see many who are still in the midst of the infertility struggle. We see some who are wrestling with the terms *childfree* and *childless*. And, we're also accompanied by those simply interested in infertility joining us on the road at this time. Why are we all together as opposed to taking our various paths in life? Because at this crossroads, the sign above us simply says "What next?"

Stretching off into the distance are infinite paths, infinite possibilities. Not all paths are available to everyone, but there's still a huge variety of options. No matter what you have gone through, you have the opportunity to gain from your experiences, or to lament what you have not achieved. It's up to you to decide how you want to deal with what happens in your life.

Sure, what we're saying now is "pop psychology." We've been dealing with infertility for many years. We don't have any living children to show for that effort. We have every right to question our own statements. We have the right to scream out "Why, *us*, Lord?" with regard to our inability to have children, when "everyone *else* is pregnant." But what good would that do?

Alternatively, we can ask ourselves what we've gained through these years of trial and tribulation. There are many things we have lost or that will never come to us in this lifetime — that is fact, even given our efforts to change it.

So, if we cannot change things, we can try to accept them. Reinhold Niebuhr asked God for the same thing in a very famous prayer called the *Serenity Prayer*. Although most everyone knows the first four lines, here is more of it:

Serenity Prayer

God grant me the serenity,
To accept the things I cannot change,
The courage to change the things I can,
And the wisdom to know the difference.

Living one day at a time;
Enjoying one moment at a time;
Accepting hardship as a pathway to peace;
Taking, as you did, this sinful world as it is,
not as I would have it.
Trusting that you will make all things right
if I surrender to your will;
That I may be reasonably happy in this life,
And supremely happy with you forever in the next.

This prayer, written in the 1930s, or some say long before that, was adopted by Alcoholics Anonymous as a way to deal with alcoholism. Since then, it's been used to help in just about every type of crisis, although it is usually directed toward dying, grieving, and suffering.

Serenity. It is a word that encompasses peace, calm, tranquility, composure, quiet, patience, satisfaction, and reconciliation. It is indeed something to strive for when attempting to accept a situation that you cannot control. Once you are able to embrace serenity, you may even be able to go further and ask yourself, "What have I gained during my time of trial and tribulation?" Each of us will have a different answer. We need to take time to define our blessings and then start counting them. We all have blessings. We just need to focus on them.

Moving on with Your Life

In writing this book, we came to this point as well. We asked ourselves what we had gained through our journey over the years. Could we count our blessings?

- We were lucky enough to emerge from our struggle with infertility with a closer relationship and a stronger marriage. Although there were times we wanted to leave each other, we came out of this toughened, stronger, and with a greater commitment to each other.

- We have more leisure time. We do not need babysitters for a night out. We can take a vacation anywhere we want without worrying about the cost and inconvenience of children. Some parents envy us for having this time. We realized it was time to appreciate it.

- We have quiet time. We can dedicate ourselves to a goal, be it a work goal, a personal goal, or a social goal without being interrupted in that pursuit.

- We don't have to question whether or not we are good parents. We don't have to worry if we are making mistakes in the important matter of raising children.

- Our trials have made us stronger. We understand better what it feels to hurt. We can sympathize better with other people who are hurting or going through a trial in their life.

- We are more in touch with our emotions. We have developed a tougher shell to deal with life's slings and arrows.

- We have more freedom. We have more time. We have more money. We try to use these to our advantage rather than dwell on what we would have traded them for.

- We have gained an appreciation for the things we have versus what we do not have. We have learned that materialism is not one of our goals in life.

- We have gained a strong respect for silence.

- We have also gained a sense of our own mortality, and the ability to be happy through pain. These things can be a gain if you accept them as part of life.

What have you gained as you deal with or have dealt with infertility? We know this is not an easy question to answer. But you need to ask and answer that question. It is the beginning of healing, whether or not you are continuing on the path of trying to have a child.

If you are still on the road of treatments, schedules, pregnancy tests, and monthly failure, remember that you have only one life to live. It is as good or as bad as you allow it to be. How you choose to deal with your infertility will determine the quality of your life.

If you have finished the journey of infertility by having the child you desired through birth or adoption, you know you are forever changed by your experience. Look carefully so you may gain from your experiences.

If you have finished the road, and have decided to live the rest of your life without children, embrace the semantic advantage of the word *childfree* as opposed to *childless*. Know what you have gained. Otherwise, you will dwell on what you did not accomplish while expending effort to have a child.

In the end, "What next?" is *your choice*. It is a choice that depends on your attitude, demeanor, and the goals you want to realize as you move on to the next stage of your life. The quality of your life is your decision, despite what comes your way.

We wish you the absolute best as you discover your next path. We wish you happiness and success. It is your life! Choose your path wisely.

— What We've Gained —

Freedom from Chains

As I walk, I think about my life
and how it might have been.
Although I realize that is a useless task.
I cannot build on *might have beens*.
What I've gained in life comes from how I have lived
and what I have done so far.

I might have been rich and famous,
had I made other decisions.
Fame and fortune would have given me
many of the things I always desired.

I also thought I would raise children.
But, no, I did not have any.

I did find love. I found a life that many would envy.
I have been able to pursue some of my dreams
to see the world.
I play the guitar at parties.
I have close friends, some lifelong.

Even so, I sometimes discount what I've gained in life
in favor of the *might have beens*.

Although I am deep in thought, I am not alone today.
I am walking behind my friend.
He suddenly interrupts my contemplation.
I am amazed that he starts discussing a topic
which eerily echoes my own thoughts.

He says:
"You know, sometimes I wish I were someone else.
I wanted to be handsome, but I'm really quite plain.
I wanted to be a mountain climber,
but I'm obviously not fit enough.
I always wanted to play the piano.
I'd hoped to make mad, passionate love under the stars
with the love of my life."

"But, you know, despite what I never did,
I try to appreciate the things I do.
I watch the stars at night and marvel at their wonder.
I listen to birds early in the morning.
Their music is sweeter than the finest instrument.
I inhale the imagination of the human spirit
as I wander the world of black on white."

"What I do is what causes me to be me.
If I had done those other things,
I would have been a different person.
I need to make sure that, in my life,
I am satisfied that I was me."

I tell him that his perspective on life
is a breath of fresh air.
I push harder to insure his wheelchair
goes up the steep slope and into the van.
He cannot wave goodbye,
but he smiles at me
before the van takes him to the seashore.
He wants to listen to the waves and the gulls.

I return to my thoughts. Chains bind each of us.
A unique set for each individual.
They prevent us from doing or being
some of the things we wish we could do or be.
It is the size of these chains within our mind
that keeps us from appreciating our lives.

For a long time,
I have allowed the chains of desired parenthood
to be ponderously large.
The chains began as small tasks.
Over time, I allowed them to grow.
And now, with desire yet unfulfilled,
these chains have come to bind me.
I have allowed them
to prevent me from being satisfied with my life.

In my mind, I cast off as many chains as I can.
Few of them disappear.
They are large and will only go away with practice.
But it is a start. A beginning.
And one day, I plan to be free of these chains.

The *might have beens*
will always be there in the wistful halls of my mind.
But I have to live my life. I have to do what I can do.
I need to make sure that, in my life,
I am satisfied that I was me.

Notes

Afterword

Dreams die hard. In fact, we have always wondered if they ever really die. We have always believed in dreams. Dreams are what give us the energy to get up in the morning. Dreams are what drive us to greater and higher achievement in our lives.

We were taught to believe that we could achieve any dream, as long as we wanted it enough. You were probably taught the same lesson. It's pervasive. As children, we believe in our dreams. Even as adults, we are encouraged to seek those dreams.

We have sought our dream of having children for many years. But there comes a time when you realize that maybe you can't have exactly the dream you were striving for — when reality interferes and tells you to reshape your dream.

When you first realize you are infertile, reshaping the dream to include medical intervention may be enough to make the dream come true. If a couple cannot conceive together, technological advances have enabled dreams to come to fruition through donor sperm or surrogacy. For many, reshaping the "children dream" to include adoption allows a dreamer to become a parent.

We dreamed of having children, but not if it meant destroying our lives together and not being able to find happiness. We tried to fulfill our dream by spending many years on the task of having a child. In doing so, we compromised our lives and some of our happiness. Over time, we realized that we needed to go back to seeking the dreams that we had set on the back burner in the process.

We encourage you to seek your dream, but be sure that you are pursuing the dream that you truly want to pursue. Ask yourself where you are on your dream quest.

As for us, we have decided to move on with our lives. We head toward the future, to that famous "second star on the right, and straight on till morning." We have chosen a new path in our life, with different dreams and goals. We wish to travel to the limits of our reach and to seek out what meaning we can find.

It will be a grand adventure.

But, still, some dreams can never die. Even as we move on to explore the strange new world of the rest of our lives — our forever wish is, and will always be, that:

After word

"Some day, our child may meet your child."

Ode to Shawn

*The old oak has seen many a day
in the pasture, gazing upon
the visage of the countryside.*

*As a seed, it fell earthward
to this convenient spot, growing,
nurtured by the sun and rain.*

*Ah, but the seed nearby found the crack
of a city sidewalk.
And the next,
the burrow of a squirrel.*

*By what right of existence
did one flourish while others failed?
Was not the hand of God upon them all?*

*The seed, ultimate in its innocence,
fulfilled God's creation.*

*Not all are meant to live; to flourish.
But each shines as a sparkle
in the eye of the Lord.*

Dan T. Davis — 1986

From Our Children,
Who Have Gone Before Us

*We wish we could walk with you
on a cold blustery day where you'd hold us close.*

*We'd like to think you'd make hot chocolate
with marshmallows to warm our tummies.*

Pillow fights would be fun.

And whispered goodnights, knowing you were nearby.

*And when we scraped our knees,
or lost our first love,
you'd remind us that things don't always work out.*

We'd remember.

Things don't always work out, do they?

*But certain loves cannot be lost,
and knees and hearts can heal.*

*Hot chocolate can be shared in spirit,
and pillows can be used for other things.*

*And on cold blustery days,
you can still hold us close in your thoughts.*

... Good night ... **we're always nearby.**

by Shawn, Michelle, and Christy Davis as "related" to Dan T. Davis — 2001

Acknowledgements

In living the infertility journey, we found a lot to be thankful for even during times that felt unbearable.

For those couples who so generously gave of their time and stories, we want to extend a special thank you. You have blessed us with your trust to represent your personal infertility journey. Although we can't list your names, you know who you are and we are grateful. This book is a reality because of your contribution.

To our parents and siblings, we thank you for your patience and willingness to love us through the ordeal of infertility. It is appreciated.

Jan was strongly encouraged to write this book by some very special optimistic people: Carolyn Young, Nita Leininger, and Joanne Peak. Your listening ear helped her through many a cold and lonely day.

Dan gives special thanks and many dog bones to Akiko, his very empathic Sheltie. She knew just when he needed doggie hugs during those very tough to write book sections.

Finally, heartfelt thanks, love, and hugs go to all of those individuals who made this book possible. Through the many drafts of the front cover to the edits on every word in the text, we indeed received expert help. Please know that we sincerely realize we could not have made this book a reality without you.

And, to all of you reading this, we send yet one more thank you for allowing us into a very private part of your lives. We hope we have helped you in some way as well.

About the Authors

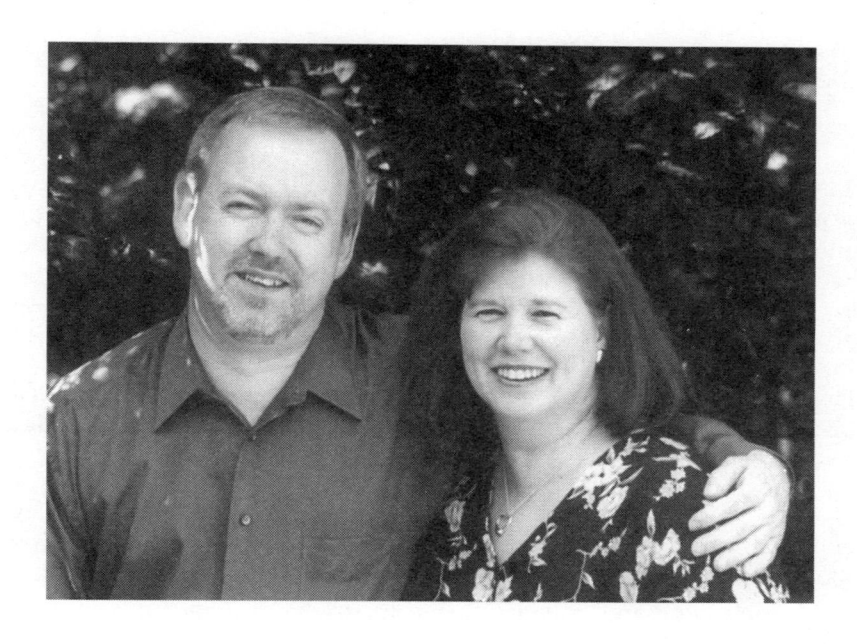

Janet L. Lazo-Davis is President of Second Star Creations, a consulting and publishing company founded in 1998. She graduated with a Masters degree from South Dakota State University and has managed an environmental engineering lab and a counseling center focusing on women with problem pregnancies. She also renovates homes for resale. Her hobbies include writing, quilting, and gardening.

Dan T. Davis helps companies build new technology businesses. His background includes time at Procter & Gamble, Universal Tax Systems, and Hallmark Cards. He graduated from the University of Florida with a Bachelor's Degree in Systems Engineering; he received two Master's Degrees at Stanford University, one in Industrial Engineering and one in Operations Research.

About Second Star Creations

Is this the last page in the book?
If so, that means the order form has been removed. But that's ok!

Just go to http://www.secondstar.us and you'll get all the information you need about how to order *Infertility's Anguish* as well as obtain the most up-to-date information about other books, projects, and activities we are working on.

If you want to go directly to information about this book instead of the Second Star Creations site, go to http://www.infertilitysanguish.com.

What is Second Star Creations?

Second Star Creations is our venture into the rest of our lives. It is a publishing company, a consulting company, and a representation of how we are now in the business of:

Turning dreams into reality

Although we were unable to have children, we have a purpose: a company to enable people to achieve their dreams — whether it is to create a business, write a book, or to simply accomplish something they have been meaning to do, but have never found the time to complete.

It is a grand adventure.

Second Star Creations

http://www.secondstar.us

Order Form

How to obtain *Infertility's Anguish*:

Best way: Go to:　　　http://www.secondstar.us

Email orders:　　　　ordersIA@secondstar.us

Postal Orders:　　　　Send this form to:
　　　　　　　　　　　Second Star Creations
　　　　　　　　　　　12120 State Line Rd #190
　　　　　　　　　　　Leawood, KS 66209-1254

Other Ways to Order:　Check website listed above.

U.S. Orders:
$17.95 per book
Add $ 3 shipping/handling for first book, $ 1 for each additional book.
Kansas residents, please add 7.525 % sales tax.

Outside U.S. or want faster delivery?
Send e-mail or check web site for total charges.

Please print clearly.

Send me _____ copies of: ***Infertility's Anguish***.

Name: _____

Address: _____

City/State/Zip: _____

Phone: _____

E-mail: _____

My check or money order in the amount of $_____ payable to *Second Star Creations* is enclosed. (U.S. funds only)

Charge my Visa or Mastercard — #_____

Expiration Date _____ Signature _____

Feel free to tear out and/or make multiple copies of this page!